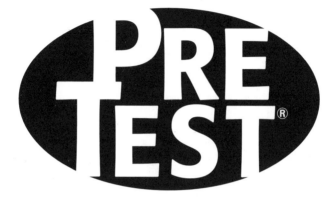

# Neuroscience

PreTest® Self-Assessment and Review

# NOTICE

Medicine is an ever-changing science. As new research and clinical experience broaden our knowledge, changes in treatment and drug therapy are required. The editors and the publisher of this work have checked with sources believed to be reliable in their efforts to provide information that is complete and generally in accord with the standards accepted at the time of publication. However, in view of the possibility of human error or changes in medical sciences, neither the editors nor the publisher nor any other party who has been involved in the preparation or publication of this work warrants that the information contained herein is in every respect accurate or complete and they are not responsible for any errors or omissions or for the results obtained from use of such information. Readers are encouraged to confirm the information contained herein with other sources. For example and in particular, readers are advised to check the product information sheet included in the package of each drug they plan to administer to be certain that the information contained in this book is accurate and that changes have not been made in the recommended dose or in the contraindications for administration. This recommendation is of particular importance in connection with new or infrequently used drugs.

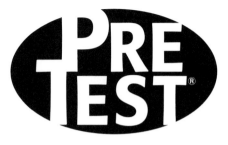

# Neuroscience
## PreTest® Self-Assessment and Review
### Third Edition

EDITED BY

**ALLAN SIEGEL, PH.D.**

Department of Neuroscience
New Jersey Medical School
Newark, New Jersey
and

**HEIDI SIEGEL, M.D.**

Epilepsy Research Branch
National Institute of Neurological Disorders and Stroke
National Institute of Health
Bethesda, Maryland

STUDENT REVIEWERS

**R. HENRY CAPPS, JR.**

East Carolina University School of Medicine
Greenville, North Carolina

**PAMELA JASMINE SCHUTZER**

Albany Medical College
Albany, New York

 **McGraw-Hill**
**Health Professions Division**
**PreTest® Series**

NEW YORK   ST. LOUIS   SAN FRANCISCO   AUCKLAND
BOGOTÁ   CARACAS   LISBON   LONDON   MADRID
MEXICO CITY   MILAN   MONTREAL   NEW DELHI
SAN JUAN   SINGAPORE   SYDNEY   TOKYO   TORONTO

# McGraw-Hill

*A Division of The McGraw·Hill Companies*

1 2 3 4 5 6 7 8 9 0   DOCDOC   9 9 8

**ISBN 0-07-052690-7**

*The editors were John Dolan, Susan Noujaim, and Deborah L. Harvey.*
*The editing supervisor was Peter McCurdy.*
*The production supervisor was Helene G. Landers.*
*The text designer was Jim Sullivan/RepoCat Graphics & Editorial Services.*
*The cover designer was Li Chen Chang/Pinpoint.*
*This book was set in Berkeley Book by Joanne Morbit of McGraw-Hill's Professional Book Group composition unit, Hightstown, NJ.*
*R.R. Donnelley & Sons was printer and binder.*

*This book is printed on acid-free paper.*

*To Carla, wife and mother,*
*whose patience, support and understanding*
*made this book possible*
*and*
*To David and Jennifer*

# CONTENTS

## THE BRAINSTEM AND CRANIAL NERVES

## SENSORY SYSTEMS

## ANATOMY OF THE FOREBRAIN

## MOTOR SYSTEMS

## HIGHER FUNCTIONS

## CLINICAL CASES

# PREFACE

The study of the neurosciences has undergone remarkable growth over the past two decades. To a large extent, such advancements have been made possible through the development of new methodologies, especially in the fields of neuropharmacology, molecular biology, and neuroanatomy. Neuroscience courses presented in medical schools and related schools of health professions generally are unable to cover all the material that has evolved in recent years. For this reason, Neuroscience: PreTest® SelfAssessment and Review was written for medical students preparing for licensing examinations as well as for undergraduate students in the health professions.

The subject matter of this book is mainly anatomy and physiology of the nervous system. Also, an attempt was made to encompass the subjects of molecular and biophysical properties of membranes, neuropharmacology, and higher functions of the nervous system. Moreover, clinical correlations for each part of the central nervous system, often using MRI and CT scans, are presented. While it is virtually impossible to cover all aspects of neuroscience, the objective of this book is to include its most significant components as we currently understand them.

The authors wish to express their gratitude to Leo Wolansky, M.D., and Alan Zimmer, M.D. for providing the MRI and CT scans.

# INTRODUCTION

Each *PreTest® Self-Assessment and Review* allows medical students to comprehensively and conveniently assess and review their knowledge of a particular basic science, in this instance Neuroscience. The 500 questions parallel the format and degree of difficulty of the questions found in the United States Medical Licensing Examination (USMLE) Step 1. Practicing physicians who want to hone their skills before USMLE Step 3 or recertification may find this to be a good beginning in their review process.

Each question is accompanied by an answer, a paragraph explanation, and a specific page reference to an appropriate textbook or journal article. A bibliography listing sources can be found following the last chapter of this text.

An effective way to use this PreTest is to allow yourself one minute to answer each question in a given chapter. As you proceed, indicate your answer beside each question. By following this suggestion, you approximate the time limits imposed by the Step.

After you finish going through the questions in the section, spend as much time as you need verifying your answers and carefully reading the explanations provided. Pay special attention to the explanations for the questions you answered incorrectly—but read *every* explanation. The authors of this material have designed the explanations to reinforce and supplement the information tested by the questions. If you feel you need further information about the material covered, consult and study the references indicated.

The High-Yield Facts added for this third edition are condensed summaries and are provided to facilitate rapid review of Neuroscience topics. It is anticipated that the reader will use the High-Yield Facts as a "memory jog" before proceeding through the questions.

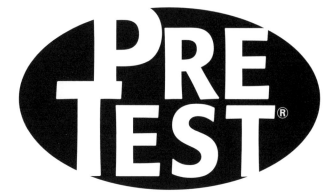

# Neuroscience

PreTest® Self-Assessment and Review

# GROSS ANATOMY
## OF THE BRAIN

## *Questions*

**DIRECTIONS:** Each group of questions below consists of lettered points on a figure followed by a set of numbered items. For each numbered item select the **one** lettered point on the figure with which it is **most** closely associated. Each lettered point may be used **once, more than once, or not at all.**

**Questions 1–7**

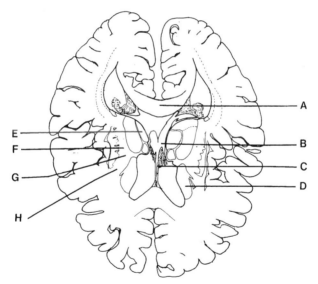

(Adapted from DeArmond et al., Fig. 15; with permission.)

**1.** This area contains fibers that arise from the leg region of the precentral gyrus.

**2.** This region contains fibers that project primarily if not exclusively to the pons.

**3.** A lesion at this site could produce weakness of muscles that mediate swallowing, chewing, breathing, and speaking.

**4.** Fibers in this region project to the mamillary bodies.

**5.** This structure is a major receiving area of the basal ganglia for afferent fibers arising from the cerebral cortex.

**6.** This structure has extensive projections to the rostral aspect of the frontal lobe, including the prefrontal cortex.

**7.** This region receives major dopaminergic inputs from the substantia nigra.

## Questions 8–15

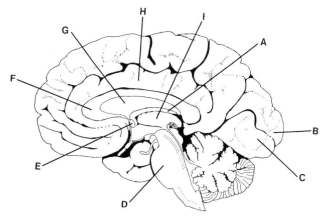

(Adapted from DeArmond et al., Fig. 4; with permission.)

**8.** This commissure of the brain conveys olfactory information.

**9.** This structure forms the medial wall of the lateral ventricle.

**10.** This cortical structure is considered part of the limbic lobe and receives a significant input from the anteroventral thalamic nucleus.

**11.** Loss of cells in this region results in loss of vision in the lower visual field.

**12.** This bundle constitutes a major fiber pathway of the hippocampal formation.

**13.** Cells in this region constitute the second-order neurons of a fiber pathway from the cerebral cortex to the cerebellar cortex.

**14.** Damage to this region unilaterally will produce an upper quadrantanopia.

**15.** Communication between the frontal lobes of each side of the brain is mediated through this structure.

## Questions 16–24

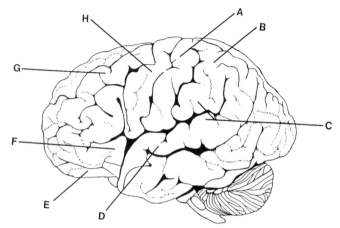

(Adapted from DeArmond et al., Fig. 10-2; with permission.)

**16.** Cells in this region give rise to fibers that supply the cervical cord.

**17.** This region receives somatosensory inputs from the lower limb.

**18.** A lesion of this region will likely result in "receptive" aphasia.

**19.** This region receives auditory inputs from the medial geniculate nucleus.

**20.** A lesion at this site will produce a speech deficit referred to as "expressive" aphasia.

**21.** This region of the brain is associated with higher intellectual functions.

**22.** This region of cortex sends significant projections to the pretectal region and superior colliculus.

**23.** A lesion of this region will typically produce a disorder involving negligence of the opposite body half and visual space.

**24.** A lesion at this site would typically produce an upper motor neuron paralysis.

## Questions 25–35

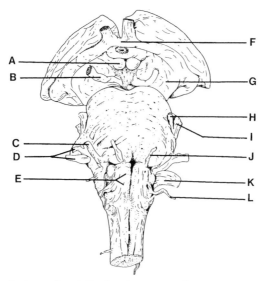

(Adapted from DeArmond et al., Fig. 6; with permission.)

**25.** This fiber bundle contains axons from neurons in the nucleus ambiguus.

**26.** This structure controls muscles of mastication.

**27.** The axons from neurons in this structure project to the anteroventral thalamic nucleus.

**28.** This nerve controls the muscles of facial expression.

**29.** Fibers in this region may terminate in the midbrain, pons, medulla, or spinal cord.

**30.** First-order neurons from this area mediate somatosensory signals from the face.

**31.** Damage to this structure could produce both a medial gaze paralysis and failure of pupillary constriction.

**32.** Damage to this structure produces a lateral gaze paralysis.

**33.** Disruption of fibers at this site resulting from a tumor would likely produce a bitemporal hemianopsia.

**34.** These fibers mediate impulses that signal changes in the position of the head.

**35.** A lesion of this nerve will cause the tongue to deviate to the side of the lesion.

**DIRECTIONS:** Each question or incomplete statement below contains five suggested responses. Select the **one best** response.

**36.** The walls that form the cisterns encasing the brain include

a. Ependyma and nerve cells
b. Dura mater and ependyma
c. Pia mater and arachnoid
d. Arachnoid and ependyma
e. Pia mater, arachnoid, and dura mater

**37.** Which of the following statements about the blood-brain barrier is correct?

a. It has well-developed capillary pores that allow for selective diffusion of substances
b. It is selectively permeable to certain compounds such as biogenic amines
c. It is found within all structures enclosed by the meninges, including the pineal gland
d. Tight junctions associated with the blood-brain barrier are formed exclusively by neuronal or glial processes
e. The blood-brain barrier is generally limited to highly vascular regions of the brain such as those present at the level of the ventromedial hypothalamus

# GROSS ANATOMY OF THE BRAIN

## *Answers*

**1–7. The answers are: 1-f, 2-h, 3-g, 4-b, 5-d, 6-e, 7-d.** (*Nolte, 3/e, pp 252–259, 261–264, 307–312, 374–378.*) This figure is a horizontal view of the brain at the level of the head of the caudate nucleus and the internal capsule. The posterior limb of the internal capsule (F) contains fibers that arise from the leg region of cerebral cortex and project to lumbar levels of spinal cord, thus serving as upper motor neurons for the elicitation of voluntary movement of the contralateral leg. Fibers in the anterior limb of the internal capsule (H) project in large numbers to deep pontine nuclei and represent first-order neurons in a pathway linking the cerebral cortex with the cerebellum. Pseudobulbar palsy is characterized in part by a weakness of the muscles controlling swallowing, chewing, breathing, and speaking. It results from a lesion of the upper motor neurons associated with the head region of the cortex, which pass through the genu of the internal capsule (G) en route to brainstem cranial nerve nuclei upon which they synapse. The descending column of the fornix (B), situated along the midline of the brain, contains fibers that arise from the hippocampal formation and project in large part to the mamillary bodies.

The head of the caudate nucleus (D) is part of an important element of the motor systems called the basal ganglia. It receives significant inputs from several regions associated with motor functions. These include the cerebral cortex and the dopamine-containing region of the substantia nigra (i.e., pars compacta). The mediodorsal thalamic nucleus (E) projects large quantities of axons to extensive regions of the rostral half of the frontal lobe, including the prefrontal cortex. It also receives significant projections from the prefrontal region of cortex.

**8–15. The answers are: 8-e, 9-g, 10-h, 11-b, 12-a, 13-d, 14-c, 15-f.** (*Nolte, 3/e, pp 27–31, 252–259, 266–268, 288–297, 300–303, 346–347, 367–370, 371–373, 394–396, 397–409.*) This figure is a midsagittal section of the brain. A major portion of the anterior commissure (E) contains fibers that arise from the olfactory bulb and decussate to the contralateral olfactory bulb. The septum pellucidum (G) forms the medial wall of the lateral ventricle, which in fact separates the lateral ventricle on one side from that on the opposite side. The cingulate gyrus (H) is a prominent structure on the medial aspect of the cerebral cortex and constitutes a component of the limbic lobe. It receives a significant input from the anteroventral thalamic nucleus.

The major output pathway of the hippocampal formation is the fornix system of fibers (A), which arise from cells in its subicular cortex and adjoining regions of hippocampus. These fibers are then distributed to the anterior thalamic nucleus, mamillary bodies, and septal area. The basilar portion of the pons (D) lies in the ventral half of this region of brainstem. It receives inputs from each of the lobes of the cerebral cortex, which it then relays to the cerebellar cortex. The primary visual cortex lies on both banks of the calcarine fissure. Cells located on the lower bank receive inputs from the lateral geniculate nucleus that relate to either the nasal or temporal upper visual fields. Therefore, a lesion of this region would produce an upper quadrantanopia (i.e., loss of one quarter of the visual field). The corpus callosum constitutes the major channel by which the cerebral cortex on one side can communicate with the cortex of the opposite side. The genu of the corpus callosum (F) contain fibers that pass from the frontal lobe of one side to that of the other.

**16–24. The answers are: 16-h, 17-a, 18-c, 19-d, 20-f, 21-e, 22-g, 23-b, 24-h.** (*Nolte, 3/e, pp 19–23, 48–52, 246–249, 266–269, 311–313, 383–385.*) This figure is a lateral view of the cerebral cortex. Cells in the "arm" area of the primary motor cortex (H) project their axons to the cervical level of the spinal cord. This area receives major input from the ventrolateral nucleus of the thalamus. The "leg" region of the primary somatosensory cortex (A) lies immediately caudal to the central sulcus, is almost devoid of pyramidal cells, and is referred to as a "granulous" cortex. Damage to the cells situated in the region of the dorsal border of the superior temporal gyrus and adjoining area of the inferior parietal lobule (Wernicke's area) (C) cause impairment in the appreciation of the meanings of written or spoken words.

The primary, secondary, and tertiary auditory receiving areas in the cortex are located mainly in the superior temporal gyrus (D). It is the final receiving area for inputs from the medial geniculate nucleus, which represents an important relay in the transmission of auditory signals to the cortex.

An additional area of the cortex governing speech (F) is called the *motor speech area*, or *Broca's area*. It is situated in the inferior aspect of the frontal lobe immediately rostral and slightly ventral to the precentral gyrus. Lesions of this region produce impairment of ability to express words in a meaningful way or to use words correctly. The orbital frontal cortex (E) lies in a position inferior and rostral to Broca's motor speech area. This region governs higher-order intellectual functions and some aspects of emotional behavior.

The caudal aspect of the middle frontal gyrus (G) contains cells that, when activated, produce conjugate deviation of the eyes. This action is believed to be accomplished, in part, by virtue of descending projections to the superior colliculus, pretectal region, and horizontal gaze center of the pons. Lesions of the posterior parietal lobe (B) of the nondominant hemisphere will produce a disorder of body image referred to as "sensory neglect." The patient will frequently fail to recognize or neglect to shave or wash those body parts. The patient may even fail to recognize the presence of a hemiparesis involving that part of the body as well. The precentral gyrus (H) constitutes the primary motor cortex. Lesions of this region produce an upper motor neuron paralysis involving a contralateral limb.

**25–35. The answers are: 25-k, 26-h, 27-a, 28-c, 29-g, 30-i, 31-b, 32-j, 33-f, 34-d, 35-l.** (*Nolte, 3/e, pp 154–174, 176–198.*) This figure is a ventral view of the brainstem. Fibers that arise from the nucleus ambiguus exit the brain on the lateral side of the medulla as part of the vagus nerve (K) and innervate the muscles of the larynx and pharynx as special visceral efferents. The motor root (H) lies medial to the sensory root and innervates the muscles of mastication. The mamillary bodies (A), which lie on the ventral surface of the brain at the caudal aspect of the hypothalamus, project many of their axons to the anteroventral thalamic nucleus as the mamillothalamic tract. The facial nerve (C) exits the brain at the level of the ventrolateral aspect of the caudal pons and its special visceral efferent component innervates the muscles of facial expression.

The cerebral peduncle (G) is situated in the ventrolateral aspect of the midbrain and contains fibers of cortical origin that project to all levels of the neuraxis of the brainstem and spinal cord. Note that the selection of choice E, the pyramids, would not have been a correct choice since the fibers present at this level can only terminate within the medulla or spinal cord. First-order somatosensory fibers from the region of the face (I) enter the brain laterally at the level of the middle of the pons as the sensory root of the trigeminal nerve. The oculomotor nerve (B) exits the brain at the level of the ventromedial aspect of the midbrain and some fibers of the general somatic efferent component of this nerve innervate the medial rectus. Damage to this component results in a loss of ability for medial gaze. Another component of the oculomotor nerve, the GVE component, constitutes the preganglionic parasympathetic neuron in a disynaptic pathway whose postganglionic division innervates the pupillary constrictor muscles. Accordingly, damage to the preganglionic division results in loss of pupillary constriction, which normally occurs in the presence of light as well as in accommodation. The abducens nerve (J) exits the brain at a ventromedial position at the level of the medullapontine border and its fibers innervate the lateral rectus muscle. Damage to this nerve results in a lateral gaze paralysis.

The optic chiasm (F) contains fibers that cross over to reach the lateral geniculate nucleus on the side contralateral to the retina from which they originated. Such fibers are associated with the temporal (i.e., lateral) visual fields. Therefore, damage to the optic chiasm will cause blindness in the lateral half of each of the visual fields. Such a deficit is referred to as *bitemporal hemianopsia.* First-order neurons from the labyrinth organs (i.e., semicircular canals, saccule, and utricle) convey information concerning the position of the head in space along the vestibular component of the eighth nerve into the central nervous system. This nerve enters the brain laterally at the level of the upper medulla. The hypoglossal nerve (L) exits the brain at the level of the middle of the medulla between the pyramid and the olive. These fibers innervate muscles that move the tongue toward the opposite side. For this reason, a lesion of the hypoglossal nucleus or its nerve will result in a deviation of the tongue to the side of the lesion because of the unopposed action of the contralateral hypoglossal nerve, which remains intact.

**36. The answer is c.** (*Nolte, 3/e, pp 33–47, 54–58.*) The meninges of the brain include pia mater, arachnoid, and dura mater. Pia mater and arachnoid are situated closest to the brain and dura mater is in an external position. Normally, the space between the pia and arachnoid is called subarachnoid space and is filled with cerebrospinal fluid. Surrounding the brain, the subarachnoid space shows local variations. At places where bulges are present, they are referred to as cisterns.

**37. The answer is b.** (*Kandel, 3/e, pp 1054–1056. Nolte, 3/e, pp 85–89.*) The blood-brain barrier is selectively permeable to certain types of substances, such as biogenic amines, and not to others. The barrier is formed by tight junctions consisting of capillary endothelial cells that are frequently in contact with the glial endfeet of astrocytes. The barrier does not contain well-developed capillary pores. It is not found within circumventricular organs such as the subfornical organ and the pineal gland but is applied to all other brain tissues.

# DEVELOPMENT

## Questions

**DIRECTIONS:** Each group of questions below consists of lettered headings followed by a set of numbered items. For each numbered item select the **one** lettered heading with which it is **most** closely associated. Each lettered heading may be used **once, more than once, or not at all.**

### Questions 38–42

Match each numbered structure with its derivation.

a. Alar plate
b. Basal plate
c. Mesencephalon
d. Rhombic lips
e. Sulcus limitans
f. Roof plate
g. Neural crest
h. Myelencephalon
i. Floor plate
j. Rathke's pouch

**38.** Alpha motor neurons

**39.** Proper sensory nucleus

**40.** Dorsal root ganglia

**41.** Spinal nucleus (cranial nerve V)

**42.** Choroid plexus

### Questions 43–46

Match each numbered structure with its derivation.

a. Neural crest cells
b. Rhombic lips
c. Mesencephalon
d. Sulcus limitans
e. Telencephalon
f. Myelencephalon
g. Floor plate
h. Rathke's pouch

**43.** Cerebellum

**44.** Amygdala

**45.** Anterior pituitary

**46.** Sympathetic ganglia

# DEVELOPMENT

## Answers

**38–42. The answers are: 38-b, 39-a, 40-g, 41-a, 42-f.** *(Noback, 5/e, pp 83–95. Nolte, 3/e, pp 6–11.)* Structures associated with motor functions, such as alpha motor neurons, are derived from the basal plate (B). Structures associated with sensory functions, such as the proper sensory nucleus and the spinal nucleus of cranial nerve V, are derived from the alar plate (A). A number of structures, such as the dorsal root ganglia, sympathetic ganglia, and chromaffin cells of the adrenal medulla, are derived from neural crest cells (G). The choroid plexus is attached to the roof of the ventricles and is thus derived from the roof plate (F).

**43–46. The answers are: 43-b, 44-e, 45-h, 46-a.** *(Noback, 5/e, pp 83–95. Nolte, 3/e, pp 6–11.)* The cerebellum is formed from the dorsolateral aspects of the alar plates, which bend medially and posteriorly to form the rhombic lips (B). The amygdala is derived from the telencephalon (E), a part of the forebrain. The anterior lobe of the pituitary is formed as an inpocket derivative of the ectodermal stomodeum called Rathke's pouch (H). The sympathetic ganglia as well as other structures (e.g., chromaffin cells of the adrenal medulla and dorsal root ganglia) are derived from neural crest cells (A).

# THE NEURON

## Questions

**DIRECTIONS:** The group of questions below consists of lettered headings followed by a set of numbered items. For each numbered item select the **one** lettered heading with which it is **most** closely associated. Each lettered heading may be used **once, more than once, or not at all.**

### Questions 47–52

The numbered items below are methods used in the anatomic or functional tracing of neurons within the nervous system. Match each method to its correct description.

a. Retrograde labeling of cell bodies
b. Immunocytochemical labeling of cell bodies
c. Labeling of sensory endings of nerve fibers
d. Labeling of receptors
e. Metabolic mapping of CNS pathways
f. Anterograde labeling of degenerating axons
g. Labeling of cell bodies and processes of neurons and glia
h. Labeling of motor nerve endings
i. Visualization of demyelination
j. Anterograde tracing of neurons in which axonal transport is utilized

**47.** Fink-Heimer methods

**48.** Horseradish peroxidase (HRP) histochemistry

**49.** Magnetic resonance imaging (MRI)

**50.** 2-Deoxyglucose autoradiography

**51.** Gold chloride method

**52.** Golgi method

**DIRECTIONS:** Each numbered question or incomplete statement below is NEGATIVELY phrased. Select the **one best** lettered response.

**53.** All the following events occur during the process of retrograde degeneration EXCEPT

a. A displacement of the nucleus toward the periphery of the cell
b. An initial swelling of the cell body
c. A proliferation of Nissl granules
d. Degeneration of processes along the axon distal to the lesion
e. An initial accumulation of mitochondria in the axoplasm at the nodes of Ranvier

**54.** All the following statements concerning myelin are true EXCEPT

a. In the peripheral nervous system, myelin is formed from Schwann cells
b. The plasmalemma of the Schwann cell surrounds an axon and spirals around the axon in concentric layers
c. The spaces between Schwann cells will become nodes of Ranvier
d. The same group of proteins are found in myelin of both the central and peripheral nervous systems
e. In oligodendrocytes the genes that encode myelin are "turned on" by the presence of axons

**55.** All the following statements about nerve cells are true EXCEPT

a. Messenger RNA molecules for cytosolic proteins emerge from the nuclear pores and become associated with ribosomes to form free polysomes in the cytoplasm
b. Cytosolic proteins show little modification or processing following their translation
c. Secretory proteins undergo little or no modification or processing after translation
d. Nuclear and mitochondrial proteins that are encoded by the cell's nucleus are targeted to their proper organelle by a process called *post-translational importation*
e. More than one copy of the same peptide as well as different peptides may be cut from the same precursor molecule

**56.** All the following statements concerning axoplasmic transport are correct EXCEPT

a. Evidence suggests it is not likely that microtubules are involved in the retrograde transport of particles
b. There exists a slow transport system that involves the movement of soluble enzymes and proteins
c. There exists a fast transport system that involves the movement of newly synthesized membranous organelles within the axon
d. A considerable percentage of the material transported consists of synaptic vesicles or their precursors destined for the axon terminals
e. Fast axoplasmic transport has been shown to have bidirectional movement (in both anterograde and retrograde directions)

**57.** All the following are likely to be involved in the gating of channels EXCEPT

a. Binding of a ligand to its receptor
b. Continuous exposure to a high concentration of a given ligand
c. Protein phosphorylation and dephosphorylation
d. Mechanical force that stretches the membrane
e. Conformational changes in the channel proteins

**58.** All the following statements concerning ion channels are correct EXCEPT

a. The ion flux through ion channels is generally regarded as a highly active process that requires the expenditure of metabolic energy
b. Most cation channels are selective in that they are permeable to a single type of ion
c. Ion flow is normally characterized by the nature of the voltage dependence of the channel's conductance
d. The electrochemical driving force is determined by the electrical potential difference and the chemical concentration gradient of the ions across the membrane
e. Ionic flow through a single channel saturates at higher concentrations of that ion

**59.** All the following statements concerning membrane potential are true EXCEPT

a. The resting membrane potential is directly proportional to separation of charge across the membrane
b. A membrane is depolarized when the separation of charge across the membrane is reduced
c. As the inside of the cell is made more negative with respect to the outside, the cell becomes depolarized
d. In a cell whose membrane possesses only $K^+$ channels, the membrane potential will approach the $K^+$ equilibrium potential
e. Passive fluxes of $Na^+$ and $K^+$ are balanced by an active pump that derives energy from enzymatic hydrolysis of ATP

**60.** All the following statements concerning length constants are true EXCEPT

a. Length constant is the distance along a dendrite where the change in membrane potential produced by a current decays to approximately one third of its original value
b. Length constant increases as the membrane resistance decreases
c. Length constant decreases as the axial resistance increases
d. Length constant is greater in myelinated than in unmyelinated fibers
e. As the length constant increases in a postsynaptic neuron, the efficiency of electrotonic conduction of synaptic potentials (at that synapse) also increases

**DIRECTIONS:** Each question below contains five suggested responses. Select the **one best** response to each question.

**61.** Which of the following statements concerning ligand-gating of neuronal membrane channels is true?

a. The normal triggering mechanism for gating involves nonspecific binding by large classes of molecules
b. Channels are opened when a given molecule selectively binds with the gating molecule
c. Ligand-gating is triggered by changes in the electrical potential across the membrane
d. The channels are constructed of a mixture of proteins and lipids
e. The gating molecule shows no conformational change during the gating process

**62.** After the occurrence of an action potential, there is a repolarization of the membrane. The principal explanation for this event is that

a. Potassium channels have been opened
b. Sodium channels have been opened
c. Potassium channels have been inactivated
d. The membrane becomes impermeable to all ions
e. There has been a sudden influx of calcium

**63.** During an in vitro experiment, the membrane potential of a nerve cell is hyperpolarized to −120 mV. At that time, a transmitter, known to be inhibitory in function, is applied to the preparation and results in a depolarization of the membrane. The most likely reason for this occurrence is that

a. Inhibitory transmitters normally depolarize the postsynaptic membrane
b. The normal response of the postsynaptic membrane to any transmitter is depolarization
c. The inhibitory transmitter activates ligand-gated potassium channels
d. Sodium channels become inactivated
e. Calcium channels become activated

**Questions 64–71**

Kuffler studied the electrophysiology of glial cells, using the optic nerve and its surrounding glial sheath. He found that the mean value of the resting potential of these cells, as recorded by intracellular microelectrodes, was −89.6 mV. The potassium concentration in the bathing solution was 3 meq/L. Assume that RT/F = 61.

**64.** Assuming that the resting potential is equivalent to the potassium equilibrium potential, calculate the approximate intracellular potassium concentration (in meq/L).

a. 11
b. 33
c. 88
d. 140
e. 155

**65.** What would be the concentration of potassium (meq/L) in the bathing fluid in order to depolarize the membrane potential to zero?

a. 11
b. 33
c. 88
d. 140
e. 155

**66.** A probable explanation for the depolarization of glial cells following stimulation of nerve fibers is that it is a result of

a. A delayed increase in potassium conductance
b. An early sodium influx
c. A large efflux of sodium ions
d. A temporal summation that results in a long-lasting depolarization
e. An influx of chloride ions

**67.** Stimulation of the optic nerve with a volley of impulses caused a slow and long-lasting depolarization of the associated glial cells. The mean value of the depolarization was 12.1 mV. If this depolarization was due solely to an increase in potassium ion concentration in the intracellular clefts, calculate the change in the concentration of potassium in the extracellular environment (in meq/L).

a. 1.79
b. 36.30
c. 137.00
d. 140.50
e. $5.35 \times 10^{-6}$

**68.** The trigger zone that integrates incoming signals from other cells and initiates the signal that the neuron sends to another neuron or muscle cell is the

a. Cell body
b. Dendritic trunk
c. Dendritic spines
d. Axon hillock and initial segment
e. Axon trunk

**69.** Which of the following statements concerning the membrane time constant is correct?

a. The time constant is a function of the membrane's resistance and capacitance
b. The time constant is unrelated to the membrane's capacitance
c. The time course of the rising phase of a synaptic potential is specifically dependent upon the time constant for that cell
d. The falling phase of a synaptic potential is dependent upon active and passive membrane properties
e. The integration of synaptic potentials is unrelated to the length of the time constant

**70.** Which of the following statements concerning sodium channels is true?

a. They are opened when the membrane is hyperpolarized
b. They display a high conductance in the resting membrane
c. They open rapidly following depolarization of the membrane
d. They are rapidly inactivated by tetraethylammonium
e. They are rapidly activated by tetrodotoxin

**71.** The equilibrium potential for potassium, as determined by the Nernst equation, differs from the resting potential of the neuron because

a. An active sodium-potassium pump makes an important contribution to the regulation of the resting potential
b. The membrane is permeable to ions other than potassium
c. The Nernst equation basically considers only the relative distribution of potassium ions across the membrane
d. The resting potential is basically dependent upon the concentration of sodium but not potassium ions across the membrane
e. The Nernst equation fails to account for local changes in temperature that influence the resting membrane potential

# THE NEURON

## Answers

**47–52. The answers are: 47-f, 48-a, 49-i, 50-e, 51-h, 52-g.** (*Carpenter, 8/e, pp 87–92. Nolte, 3/e, pp 2–7, 22–23.*) The Fink-Heimer technique was used for a number of years as the method of choice for the anterograde tracing of degenerating axons from the site where the lesion was placed to the terminal endings of the damaged axons (F). In this method, the selective silver impregnation of degenerating axons permits visualization of the axons in question. With HRP histochemistry, the glycoprotein enzyme horseradish peroxidase is injected into the region of the terminal endings of the neuronal pathway under examination and is incorporated into the axons through a process of micropinocytosis. HRP is then retrogradely transported back to the cell bodies of origin of that pathway (A), where it is then degraded. By reacting the tissue with an appropriate substrate, the labeled cells can be visualized under light microscopy. MRI permits the visualization of the degenerative process that results in demyelination of axons (I). 2-Deoxyglucose (2-DG) autoradiography is used to metabolically map (E) pathways and structures that are functionally active as a result of sensory, chemical, or electrical stimulation of nervous tissue. Local variations in energy metabolism can be visualized because the glucose analogue $^{14}$C-2-deoxyglucose (2DG) is phosphorylated to 2-DG-6phosphate where it is not further metabolized and is retained in the neuron. The rate of incorporation into neurons is related to the rate of glucose utilization, which is, itself, a function of energy metabolism. The gold chloride method is a histochemical procedure that can be used for visualizing motor nerve endings in skeletal muscle (H). In this method, tissues are placed into a silver-protein solution in which the silver is reduced. When the tissue is passed through a solution of gold chloride, the gold replaces the silver particles in the nerve tissue of that section of tissue. Nonneural gold particles are removed by treatment with oxalic acid. The Golgi silver method has been widely used to visualize individual neurons and glia (G). It fills the neuron (or glial cell) with a black deposit that extends to the dendrites and axon, thus enabling the observer to clearly characterize the morphologic properties of these neurons.

**53. The answer is c.** *(Nolte, 3/e, pp 4–5.)* A number of changes occur in the neuron during the process of retrograde degeneration. The cell body initially shows some swelling and becomes distended. At the beginning of the degenerative process, there is an accumulation of mitochondria in the axoplasm at the nodes of Ranvier. The nucleus is then displaced toward the periphery of the cell. The Nissl granules break down, first in the center of the cell; later, the breakdown spreads outward. In addition, the axonal process distal to the site of the lesion will undergo degeneration. It should be noted that retrograde degeneration procedures were used experimentally prior to the advent of histochemical methods for identifying cell bodies of origin of given pathways in the CNS.

**54. The answer is e.** *(Kandel, 3/e, pp 38–44.)* In the peripheral nervous system, Schwann cells are responsible for producing myelin, while in the CNS, this function is carried out by oligodendrocytes. The myelin present along nerve fibers in both the peripheral and central nervous systems contains the same group of proteins, myelin basic proteins. Myelin is formed when the plasmalemma of the Schwann cell elongates and spirals around the axon in concentric layers. The nodes of Ranvier are spaces between Schwann cells where the axon is unsheathed. One major difference between Schwann cells and oligodendrocytes is that Schwann cell genes that encode myelin are "turned on" by other Schwann cells, while the genes in oligodendrocytes that encode myelin depend upon the presence of astrocytes rather than other axons.

**55. The answer is c.** *(Kandel, 3/e, pp 49–56.)* Cytosolic proteins are the most extensive type of protein in the cell and include those that make up the cytoskeleton and enzymes that catalyze the different metabolic reactions of the cell. Messenger RNAs for these proteins pass through nuclear pores, become associated with ribosomes, and ultimately form free polysomes in the cytoplasm of the cell. Cytosolic proteins display little modification or processing compared with proteins that remain attached to the membranes of endoplasmic reticulum or the Golgi apparatus. Messenger RNA that encodes protein that will become a constituent of organelles or secretory products is formed on polysomes that are attached to endoplasmic reticulum. Such sheets of membrane in association with ribosomes are called *rough endoplasmic reticulum*. Secretory products typically undergo significant modification after translation. For example, neuropeptide transmitters are cleaved from polypeptide chains, in part, in the endoplasmic reticulum and the Golgi apparatus. Nuclear and mitochondrial proteins are encoded by the nucleus and are formed on free polysomes. The mechanism by which they are targeted to their proper organelle is called *posttranslational importation*. Specific receptors bind and translocate these proteins, and it is the recognition of the structural features of these proteins that allows for transport into the nucleus from the cytoplasm. In the processing of large proteins such as opioid peptides, more than one copy and different peptides are produced from the same precursor molecule. This precursor is referred to as a polyprotein because more than one active peptide is present.

**56. The answer is a.** (*Kandel, 3/e, pp 57–61. Nolte, 3/e, pp 4–5.*) Transport of materials along an axon moves in both anterograde and retrograde directions. Anterograde transport involves both fast and slow transport systems. Transport in either direction utilizes microtubules as a vehicle or track by which the particles are transported. Among the particles transported down the axon from the cell body are newly synthesized membranous organelles, including synaptic vesicles or their precursors, which ultimately reach the axon terminals.

**57. The answer is b.** (*Kandel, 3/e, pp 75–79.*) It is believed that different kinds of stimuli can function to open or close channels. For example, mechanical activation may lead to the opening of channels. Some channels (ligand-gated) are regulated by the noncovalent binding of chemical ligands such as neurotransmitters; others (electrically gated) are affected by changes in membrane voltage that cause a change in the conformation of the channel. Alternatively, relatively longlasting changes may result when second messengers bind to the channel at which time there is protein phosphorylation mediated by protein kinases. Such modification of the channel can be reversed by dephosphorylation. In contrast, when a ligand-gated channel is exposed to prolonged, high concentrations of its ligand, it tends to become "refractory" (i.e., desensitized to the presence of that ligand).

**58. The answer is a.** (*Kandel, 3/e, pp 68–79.*) Ion flux through ion channels is considered to be passive in nature and functions in the absence of any mechanism that requires energy metabolism. Cation channels are generally associated with membranes that are semipermeable to selective ions such as $Na^+$, $K^+$, or $Cl^-$. The electrochemical gradient is a function of two forces: (1) the chemical concentration gradient, which is derived from the relative differences in the distributions of ions across the membrane, and (2) the electrical potential difference between the two sides of the membrane as a function of the distribution of the ionic charges. When ions may flow through channels, current varies as a function of concentration. However, at high ionic concentration differences, a saturation phenomenon is observed that is due to resistance to flow through the channels.

**59. The answer is c.** (*Kandel, 3/e, pp 82–85.*) The potential difference across the membrane is a result of the separation of charge and is called the resting membrane potential. Accordingly, the potential difference across the membrane is a direct function of the numbers of positive and negative charges on either side of the membrane. As the separation of charge across the membrane is reduced, the membrane is said to be depolarized. Conversely, as the separation of charge is increased, the membrane becomes hyperpolarized. In the latter case, the inside of the cell is made more negative with respect to the outside. If a cell has only a single channel in its membrane (such as for $K^+$), the gradients for the other ions become irrelevant and the membrane potential will approach the equilibrium potential for the single ion ($K^+$ in this example). There is a tendency for ions to leak down their electrochemical gradients from one side of the membrane to the other. In order for there to be a steady resting membrane potential, the gradients across the membrane must be held constant. Changes in ionic gradients are avoided, in spite of the leak, by the presence of an active $Na^+/K^+$ pump (a membrane protein) that moves $Na^+$ out of the cell and at the same time brings $K^+$ into the cell. Such a pumping mechanism requires energy because it is working against the electrochemical gradients of the two ions. The energy is derived from the hydrolysis of ATP.

**60. The answer is b.** (*Kandel, 3/e, pp 97–100.*) The length constant is defined as $R_m/R_a$, where $R_m$ equals membrane resistance and $R_a$ equals axial resistance. It is the distance along a fiber where a change in membrane potential produced by a given current decays to a value of approximately one third of its original value. As can be seen from the definition, the length constant is directly proportional to the membrane resistance and inversely related to the axial resistance (i.e., the resistance of the cytoplasm within the fiber). The membrane resistance is increased significantly through the process of myelination, which thus produces an increase in the value of the length constant. When the length constant along a dendrite is relatively large, it has the effect of increasing the efficiency of electrotonic conduction along the dendritic process as compared with a similar dendrite with a smaller length constant. In this manner, the synaptic potential along the dendrite distal to the synapse will be relatively larger in a dendrite that has a larger length constant than one that has a smaller length constant.

**61. The answer is b.** (*Guyton, 2/e, pp 60–61. Kandel, 3/e, pp 67–79.*) The triggering mechanism for ligand-gating involves the selective binding of a particular molecule with the protein channel. This binding causes a conformational change of the channel protein that results in the movement of the channel back and forth which, in effect, opens or closes the channel. Neurotransmitters can regulate channels as a result of their binding properties. An example is the action of acetylcholine at the neuromuscular junction, which is capable of activating channels in the membrane of skeletal muscle. Most cation channels are selective for sodium, potassium, or calcium. Ion channels are composed of large membrane glycoproteins that vary widely in their molecular weights. In contrast to ligand-gating, other types of channels may be activated by changes in the electrical potential across the cell membrane, a process referred to as "voltage-gating."

**62. The answer is a.** (*Kandel, 3/e, pp 105–118.*) In the late phase of the action potential, potassium channels become opened and potassium efflux produces a hyperpolarization of the membrane. During the repolarization of the membrane, sodium channels are closed (sodium inactivation). Recall that activation of sodium channels is associated with the generation of the action potential. Calcium has a strong electrochemical gradient that drives it into the cell; this coincides with the upstroke of the action potential. A number of different types of calcium-gated potassium channels have been described that are activated during the action potential. Thus, it would appear that calcium influx during the action potential could generate opposing effects. On the one hand, calcium influx carries a positive charge into the cell, which contributes to the depolarization of the membrane. On the other hand, calcium influx may help to open up more potassium channels, which contributes to an outward ionic flow of potassium that causes repolarization of the membrane.

**63. The answer is c.** *(Kandel, 3/e, pp 88–91, 96–102.)* To understand how an inhibitory transmitter can actually cause a partial depolarization of the membrane, refer to the Goldman equation. The release (or application) of an inhibitory transmitter will serve to open specific ion channels, notably those of potassium. If the membrane is artificially hyperpolarized to $-120$ mV, the opening of the potassium channel will lead to a redistribution of the ions across the membrane to a normal level. If the normal equilibrium potential for potassium is approximately $-75$ mV, then, application of an inhibitory transmitter (that typically functions by opening potassium channels) will result in a redistribution of potassium ions toward the potassium equilibrium potential (i.e., $-75$ mV). Consequently, the membrane potential will be reduced (i.e., depolarized) from $-120$ mV to a value close to $-75$ mV. Other possible answers are clearly incorrect. Inhibitory transmitters normally function to hyperpolarize the membrane. Postsynaptic membranes may either be depolarized or hyperpolarized, depending upon the nature of the transmitter and receptor complex present at the synapse. Since the influx of calcium during the depolarization phase of the action potential leads to opposing effects, activation of this channel cannot account for the observed effects. Inactivation of sodium channels would not result in a depolarization of the membrane, but, instead, may contribute to the hyperpolarization of the membrane.

**64. The answer is c.** *(Kandel, 3/e, pp 82–100.)* To solve the problem, use the Goldman equation, which reduces to the Nernst equation:

$$\text{Equilibrium potential} = (RT/F) \times \ln [K_i] / [K_o]$$
$$-89.6 = 61 (\ln [K_i] 2 \ln [3])$$
$$-89.6/61 = \ln [K_i] 2\ 0.48$$
$$1.47 = \ln [K_i] 2\ 0.48$$
$$1.95 = \ln [K_i]$$
$$88.54 = K_i$$

**65. The answer is c.** *(Kandel, 3/e, pp 82–100.)* If the bathing solution is brought to 88 meq/L, the ionic concentrations outside and inside the membrane would be equal and, therefore, the membrane potential would be depolarized to zero.

**66. The answer is a.** (*Kandel, 3/e, pp 82–100.*) In this situation the roles of sodium and chloride ions were not of central importance. Temporal summation also cannot account for these findings and is thus irrelevant to the question at hand. The depolarization of 12.1 mV can be attributed to an increase in the concentration of potassium in the intracellular cleft.

**67. The answer is a.** (*Kandel, 3/e, pp 82–100.*) Use the Goldman equation reduced to the Nernst equation. The resting membrane potential is $-89.6$ mV, RT/F=61, the potassium concentration is 3 meq/L, and $K_i$ is calculated to be 88.54 mV.

$$\text{Equilibrium potential} = (RT/F) \times 61 \ln (K_o/K_i)$$
$$-89.6 - 12.1 = 61 \times \ln (K_o - 88.54)$$
$$-77.5 = 61 \times (\ln K_o - \ln 88.54)$$
$$-1.27 = \ln K_o - \ln 88.54$$
$$-1.27 - (-1.95) = \ln K_o$$
$$+0.68 = \ln K_o$$
$$4.79 \text{ meq/L} = K_o$$

Therefore, the change in extracellular potassium would be:

$$4.79 - 3.00 = 1.79 \text{ meq/L}$$

**68. The answer is d.** (*Kandel, 3/e, pp 40–41.*) The trigger zone for the initiation of impulses from a neuron includes a specialized region of the cell body—the axon hillock—together with the section of the axon that adjoins this region—the initial segment. Other components of the neuron such as the dendrites and cell body receive inputs from afferent sources but are not capable of initiating impulses at these sites. The same is true concerning more distal aspects of the axon over which the impulse is conducted.

**69. The answer is a.** (*Kandel, 3/e, pp 95–97.*) The time and space constants represent passive properties of a neuron. The electrical equivalent circuit utilizes the concept that a membrane has both capacitive and resistive properties in parallel, in which case, the rising phase of a potential change is governed in part by the product of the resistance and capacitance of the membrane. The rising phase of a synaptic potential is governed by both active and passive properties of the membrane. However, the falling phase is regulated solely by the passive properties. As the time constant is increased, the probability of integration of converging synaptic signals is increased because such signals will be more likely to overlap in time (temporal summation).

**70. The answer is c.** (*Kandel, 3/e, pp 105–118.*) Sodium channels are rapidly opened following depolarization of the membrane. The rapid influx of ions results in a further depolarization of the membrane, which, in turn, can lead to an action potential. When the membrane is hyperpolarized, sodium channels are closed. Moreover, in the resting membrane, sodium channels are not activated. Tetraethylammonium is a drug that selectively blocks only potassium channels. Tetrodotoxin blocks sodium channels.

**71. The answer is b.** (*Kandel, 3/e, pp 84–86, 88–91, 100–102, 105–108.*) Because the membrane is a leaky one, the sodium-potassium pump serves an important function in actively transporting ions from one side of the membrane to the other. The membrane is permeable to ions other than potassium, such as sodium and chloride. This fact is taken into consideration in the Goldman equation. This equation includes the distribution of all of these other ions in its formula for determining the value of membrane potential. Accordingly, the resting membrane potential is dependent upon the concentration of these other ions as well as potassium. While it is true that the Nernst equation considers the relative distribution of potassium ions across the membrane, this statement, in itself, does not explain why the equilibrium potential for potassium differs from the resting potential of the neuron. The statement that the Nernst equation does not take into account differences in temperature is false. But, again, even if that statement were true, it would nevertheless not account for the differences between the equilibrium potential for potassium and the resting potential of the neuron.

# THE SYNAPSE

## Questions

**DIRECTIONS:** Each group of questions below consists of lettered headings followed by a set of numbered items. For each numbered item select the **one** lettered heading with which it is **most** closely associated. Each lettered heading may be used **once, more than once, or not at all.**

### Questions 72–77

Match each description with the appropriate potential.

a. Resting potential
b. Action potential
c. Receptor potential
d. Electrical presynaptic potentials
e. Electrical postsynaptic potentials
f. Increased-conductance presynaptic potentials
g. Increased-conductance postsynaptic potentials
h. Decreased-conductance presynaptic potentials
i. Decreased-conductance postsynaptic potentials

**72.** All or none response, approximately 100 mV

**73.** A relatively steady voltage, which varies from cell to cell and ranges from –35 to –90 mV

**74.** A graded, fast potential, lasting from several milliseconds to seconds, resulting from a chemical transmitter binding to a receptor to produce either an excitatory postsynaptic potential (EPSP) that depends upon a single class of channels for sodium and potassium or an inhibitory postsynaptic potential (IPSP) that is dependent upon chloride or potassium conductance

**75.** A graded, slow potential, lasting from seconds to minutes; contributes to the amplitude and duration of the action potential; involves a chemical transmitter and an intracellular messenger for the closure of single-ion channels

**76.** A potential that lasts for several milliseconds, is graded, and involves a single channel for both sodium and potassium ions; activated by a sensory stimulus

**77.** Passive spread to a presynaptic current across a gap junction; activated by changes in voltage, pH, or calcium ion levels

**Questions 78–81**

Match each description to the correct synapse.

a. Axodendritic synapse
b. Axoaxonic synapse
c. Axosomatic synapse
d. Somasomatic synapse
e. Dendrodendritic synapse
f. Dendroaxonic synapse
g. Dendrosomatic synapse

**78.** These synapses are frequently found to be excitatory.

**79.** These synapses are frequently found to be inhibitory.

**80.** At these synapses, the neuron is regulated as a result of the modulation of the quantity of transmitter released.

**81.** This type of synapse is characteristic of the one present between the basket and Purkinje cells of the cerebellum.

**DIRECTIONS:** Each numbered question or incomplete statement below is NEGATIVELY phrased. Select the **one best** lettered response.

**82.** All the following statements concerning chemical synapses are correct EXCEPT

a. Presynaptic terminals contain many vesicles that are normally filled with a chemical neurotransmitter
b. The postsynaptic receptor determines whether or not a transmitter will bind to a receptor molecule on the postsynaptic cell
c. The receptors are proteins
d. Receptors can provide a gating function with respect to a given ion channel
e. The mechanism of indirect gating of ions normally does not involve the activation of G proteins

**83.** Gamma-aminobutyric acid (GABA) and glycine share all the following properties EXCEPT

a. Both are known to have inhibitory as well as excitatory properties
b. Both, acting on different receptors, regulate a similar chloride channel
c. Both utilize receptors that are transmembrane proteins
d. Both have channels that produce electrical signals because ions move down their electrochemical gradients within their respective channels
e. Both are found in the spinal cord

**84.** Characteristics of the *N*-methyl-D-aspartate (NMDA) receptor include all the following EXCEPT

a. It controls a high conductance cation channel
b. The NMDA channel is easily blocked by the presence of magnesium
c. The NMDA channel has voltage-gating properties
d. Excessive amounts of glutamate, acting through NMDA receptors, may cause neuronal cell death
e. Current flow is blocked in the presence of glutamate, leading to hyperpolarization of the cell

**DIRECTIONS:**   Each question below contains five suggested responses. Select the **one best** response to each question.

**85.** Which of the following is a second messenger system directly activated by the binding of norepinephrine to a beta-adrenergic receptor?

a. Inositol 1,4,5-triphosphate ($IP_3$)
b. Cyclic AMP
c. Diacylglycerol (DAG)
d. Arachidonic acid
e. Prostaglandins

**86.** Inhibition at the synapse is governed by

a. Chloride and sodium
b. Chloride and potassium
c. Potassium and sodium
d. Sodium and calcium
e. Sodium only

**87.** The release of transmitter is directly governed by

a. Sodium influx
b. Sodium efflux
c. Potassium influx
d. Potassium efflux
e. Calcium influx

**88.** Which of the following statements is appropriate to second messengers within neurons?

a. They have little effect upon receptors
b. They can regulate gene expression that could lead to neuronal growth and the synthesis of new proteins
c. They have little effect upon the closing of ion channels
d. They have little effect upon the opening of ion channels
e. They are directly involved in the gating of sodium channels by NMDA receptors

**89.** N-methyl-D-aspartate (NMDA), kainate, and quisqualate all act on which of the following receptors?

a. Gamma-aminobutyric acid receptors
b. Excitatory amino acid receptors
c. Adrenergic receptors
d. Opioid receptors
e. Dopamine receptors

# THE SYNAPSE

## Answers

**72–77. The answers are: 72-b, 73-a, 74-g, 75-i, 76-c, 77-e.** *(Kandel, 3/e, pp 123–172.)* The action potential (B) is characterized by an all or none response in which the overshoot may reach an amplitude of up to 100 mV. The mechanism involves separate ion channels for sodium and potassium. The resting potential (A) is characterized by a relatively steady potential, usually in the region of $-70$ mV, but which may range from $-35$ to $-70$ mV. This potential is mainly dependent upon potassium and chloride channels. Increased-conductance postsynaptic potentials (G) are fast, graded potentials, lasting from several milliseconds to several seconds. If the potential is an EPSP, it depends upon a single class of ligand-gated channels for sodium and potassium. If the response is an IPSP, then it depends upon ligand-gated channels for potassium and chloride. Decreased-conductance postsynaptic potentials (I) are mediated by a chemical transmitter or intracellular messenger to produce a graded, slow potential, lasting from seconds to minutes. This response is related to a closure of sodium, potassium, or chloride channels. Receptor potentials (C) result from the application of a sensory stimulus that produces a fast, graded potential that involves a single class of channels for both sodium and potassium. Electrical postsynaptic potentials (E) involve the passive spread of current across a gap junction that is permeable to a variety of small ions. The stimulus for such activation may be a change in either voltage, pH, or intracellular calcium.

**78–81. The answers are: 78-a, 79-c, 80-b, 81-c.** *(Kandel, 3/e, pp 166–172, 626–632.)* The overwhelming number of excitatory synapses are observed to be axodendritic (A). The presynaptic axon may synapse upon either the dendritic spine or the dendritic trunk. In contrast, axon terminals that make synaptic contact with the soma (C) of postsynaptic cells are frequently observed to be inhibitory. A classic example of this is in the cerebellar cortex, where an interneuron (basket cell) makes synaptic contact with the soma of the Purkinje cell. Activation of the basket cell results in subsequent inhibition of the Purkinje cell. Axoaxonic synapses are formed when an axon terminal comes into synaptic contact with another axon. While axoaxonic synapses have no direct effect upon the trigger zone of the postsynaptic cell, they affect that cell's functioning indirectly by modulating the amount of transmitter released from its axon terminals. Dendrodendritic synapses have been identified in the olfactory bulb and have been shown to be inhibitory. They are not found with any frequency in any other region of the central nervous system.

**82. The answer is e.** *(Kandel, 3/e, pp 131–134.)* The presynaptic terminals of chemical synapses typically contain synaptic vesicles. The vesicles may be round or flat, and filled or empty. They are typically filled with a neurotransmitter that is released onto the synaptic cleft. The receptive process on the postsynaptic region—i.e., the postsynaptic receptor—takes on a very important function. The binding of the transmitter to the receptor molecule is determined by this receptor, which is a membrane-spanning protein. Perhaps the most significant feature of the receptor is that it serves a gating function for particular ions. It can do this either directly, if it is part of the ion channel, or indirectly, by activating a G protein that, in turn, activates a second messenger system. This process results in a modulation of the ion channel's activity. In particular, the G protein stimulates adenylate cyclase, converting ATP to cAMP. In turn, cAMP induces activation of cAMPdependent protein kinase, which modulates channels by phosphorylating the channel protein or some other protein that works on that channel.

**83. The answer is a.** *(Kandel, 3/e, pp 160–170.)* Both GABA and glycine are inhibitory transmitters found in the spinal cord and elsewhere in the central nervous system. Accordingly, they both act on a similar chloride channel, which, when activated, permits this ion to enter the cell and make it more negative (i.e., hyperpolarize the cell). Each of the channels is formed from a transmembrane protein. It contains a transmitter binding site on the outer side of the membrane, and its conducting pore is embedded in the cell membrane. Another feature—that both channels produce electrical signals as a result of the movement of ions down their electrochemical gradients within their channels—is a feature common to both excitatory and inhibitory transmitters.

**84. The answer is e.** *(Kandel, 3/e, pp 152–160.)* The NMDA receptor regulates a channel permeable to several cations, which include calcium, sodium, and potassium. This channel, however, is easily blocked by magnesium. In fact, it requires a significant depolarization of the membrane in order for magnesium to be exuded from the channel so that sodium and calcium can enter the cell. One of the unusual features of this transmitter-gated channel is that it is also gated by voltage. Thus, conductance reaches its peak when both glutamate is present and the cell is depolarized. High concentrations of glutamate could result in death of the cell. This may be due to an unusually large influx of calcium through NMDA-activated channels. The calcium might activate proteases, resulting in the formation of free radicals that could be toxic to the cell.

**85. The answer is b.** *(Kandel, 3/e, pp 173–176.)* When norepinephrine reaches a beta-adrenergic receptor, a G protein activates adenyl cyclase, which generates a second messenger, cyclic AMP, from ATP. Cyclic AMP activates a cyclic AMP-dependent kinase that alters the conformation of regulatory subunits of other kinases. This frees catalytic subunits to phosphorylate specific proteins, which, in turn, leads to the cellular response. $IP_3$ and DAG are associated with the transmitter acetylcholine, which binds to muscarinic receptors, and arachidonic acid is linked to histamine, which binds to histamine receptors. Prostaglandins are metabolites of arachidonic acid.

**86. The answer is b.** *(Kandel, 3/e, pp 160–168.)* In neurons within the CNS, an inhibitory transmitter will open chloride channels. In addition, second messengers may also mediate inhibition. It is likely that they do so by opening potassium channels. When a chloride channel is opened, it will lead to movement of this ion down its concentration gradient and into the cell. This will make the cell more negative (i.e., hyperpolarized). At the same time, there will be an efflux of potassium, which will also produce hyperpolarization of the cell because positive charges are now being removed. On the other hand, sodium and calcium influx are associated with depolarization of the cell.

**87. The answer is e.** *(Kandel, 3/e, pp 194–211.)* Experimental methods permit evaluation of the relative contributions of different ions in the regulation of transmitter release. Neither tetrodotoxin, which blocks voltage-gated sodium channels, nor tetraethylammonium, which blocks voltage-gated potassium channels, will block the generation of a postsynaptic potential when the presynaptic cell is artificially depolarized. In contrast, presynaptic calcium influx triggers the release of transmitter and results in a postsynaptic potential. Moreover, when presynaptic calcium influx is blocked, no postsynaptic potential is produced. Action potentials at the presynaptic axon terminals open up calcium channels, permitting calcium influx. This event helps move synaptic vesicles to active sites as actin filaments (which anchor the vesicles) are dissolved.

**88. The answer is b.** (*Kandel, 3/e, pp 180–192.*) Second messenger kinases can lead to the phosphorylation of ion channel proteins. Such a process can lead to either the closing of a previously open ion channel or opening of a previously closed channel. For example, norepinephrine acts through cyclic AMP to close the potassium channel, resulting in an increase in excitability. Second messengers can phosphorylate transcriptional regulatory proteins and thus alter gene expression. In particular, existing proteins may be altered and new proteins may be synthesized. Moreover, such effects may generate other alterations such as the induction of neuronal growth. Second messengers can also interact directly with an ion channel to cause it to open or close (in the absence of a protein kinase). They also can produce a level of desensitization in receptors, which is a function of the extent of phosphorylation. The direct gating of ion channels by NMDA receptors is an example of a process that does not immediately involve a second messenger.

**89. The answer is b.** (*Kandel, 3/e, pp 157–160.*) NMDA, kainate, and quisqualate act upon excitatory amino acid receptors. The NMDA receptor differs from the other types of receptors in that it is blocked by $Mg^{2+}$ and controls a cation channel permeable to calcium, sodium, and potassium. Pharmacologically, NMDA receptors can be blocked by 2-amino-5-phosphonovaleric acid. The quisqualate receptor is activated by quisqualic acid; it has a high affinity for L-glutamate and α-amino-hydroxy-5-methyl-4-isoxazolepropionic acid (AMPA). The kainate receptor is activated by kainic acid. It regulates a channel that is permeable to sodium and potassium, binds AMPA, and is important in the process of excitotoxicity.

# NEUROTRANSMITTERS

## Questions

**DIRECTIONS:** The questions below consist of lettered headings followed by a set of numbered items. For each numbered item select the **one** heading with which it is **most** closely associated. Each lettered heading may be used **once, more than once, or not at all.**

### Questions 90–94

Match each description with the correct substance.

a. Tyrosine
b. Dopamine β-hydroxylase
c. Dihydroxyphenylalanine (DOPA)
d. Tryptophan hydroxylase
e. Tyrosine hydroxylase
f. Tryptophan
g. Phenylalanine
h. Epinephrine
i. Melatonin

**90.** An immediate precursor of dopamine

**91.** Rate-limiting enzyme in the biosynthesis of serotonin

**92.** Amino acid precursor of DOPA

**93.** First enzyme involved in the biosynthesis of catecholamines

**94.** Enzyme that converts dopamine to norepinephrine

### Questions 95–99

Match each description with the appropriate substance.

a. Serotonin
b. p-Chlorophenylalanine
c. Dopamine
d. Norepinephrine
e. Epinephrine
f. Phenylethanolamine-N-methyl-transferase
g. Acetylcholine
h. Monoamine oxidase
i. Phenylalanine

**95.** Immediate precursor of epinephrine

**96.** Selective destruction by 5, 7-dihydroxytryptamine (5,7-DHT)

**97.** Depletion of brain serotonin

**98.** Contribution to metabolic degradation of catecholamines

**99.** Immediate precursor of norepinephrine

## Questions 100–104

Match each description with the correct substance.

a. Norepinephrine
b. Dopamine
c. Enkephalin
d. Acetylcholine
e. Somatostatin
f. Glycine
g. Glutamate
h. Gamma-aminobutyric acid (GABA)
i. Serotonin

**100.** Present in the spinal cord as an inhibitory neurotransmitter

**101.** Present in raphe neurons of the pons

**102.** Present in cortical projection neurons to the neostriatum

**103.** Present in the pars compacta of the substantia nigra

**104.** Present in high concentrations within the nucleus basalis of the rostrobasal forebrain

## Questions 105–109

Match each description with the appropriate substance.

a. Norepinephrine
b. Dopamine
c. Serotonin
d. Gamma-aminobutyric acid (GABA)
e. Enkephalins
f. Substance P
g. Somatostatin
h. Acetylcholine
i. Neuropeptide Y

**105.** Neurotransmitter present in the locus ceruleus of the pons

**106.** Factor found in high concentrations in midbrain periaqueductal gray; modulates pain impulses

**107.** Excitatory neurotransmitter released from primary afferent neuronal terminals in the dorsal horn of the spinal cord

**108.** Inhibitory neurotransmitter that is directly antagonized by biculline and benzodiazepines

**109.** Factor present in the hypothalamus; inhibits secretion of growth hormone

## Questions 110–114

Match each description with the appropriate compound.

a. Yohimbine
b. Ketanserin
c. Prazosin
d. Metoprolol
e. Sulpiride
f. Lysergic acid diethylamide (LSD)
g. Clonidine
h. Atropine
i. Amphetamine

**110.** Alpha$_1$-adrenergic receptor antagonist

**111.** Alpha$_2$-adrenergic receptor agonist

**112.** Alpha$_2$-adrenergic receptor antagonist

**113.** Beta1-adrenergic receptor antagonist

**114.** Dopamine D$_2$ receptor antagonist

## Questions 115–119

Match each description with the correct substance.

a. Substance P
b. Naloxone
c. Dynorphin
d. Oxotremorine
e. Clozapine
f. Atropine
g. Somatostatin
h. Morphine
i. Substance K

**115.** Opiate agonist at $\mu$ receptors

**116.** Opiate antagonist

**117.** Muscarinic agonist

**118.** Antagonist at serotonin$_{1C}$ and serotonin$_2$ receptors

**119.** Opiate agonist at $\kappa$ receptors

## Questions 120–122

Match each description with the correct substance.

a. Histamine
b. Serotonin
c. Vasopressin
d. Oxytocin
e. Somatostatin
f. Enkephalin

**120.** A precursor of melatonin

**121.** Confirmed presence only in the posterior hypothalamus

**122.** Promotion of water conservation

## Questions 123–126

Match each description with the correct receptor.

a. L-AP4 receptor
b. Kainate receptor
c. N-methyl-D-aspartate (NMDA) receptor
d. Alpha-amino-3-hydroxy-5-methylisoxazole-4-propionic acid (AMPA) receptor
e. $GABA_A$ receptor
f. $GABA_B$ receptor
g. Glycine receptor

**123.** A receptor activated by baclofen

**124.** A receptor that can be selectively blocked by quinoxaline-diones

**125.** A receptor that requires the simultaneous binding of two different agonists for activation

**126.** A metabotropic receptor found in the retina

**DIRECTIONS:**   Each question below contains five suggested responses. Select the **one best** response to each question.

**127.** The biochemical sequence involved in synaptic transmission is

a. Transmitter synthesis → binding of transmitter to postsynaptic receptor → release of transmitter into synaptic cleft → destruction of transmitter
b. Transmitter synthesis → release of transmitter into synaptic cleft → binding of transmitter to postsynaptic receptor → removal of transmitter
c. Transmitter synthesis → breakdown of calcium channels → binding of transmitter to postsynaptic receptor → destruction of receptor
d. Breakdown of calcium channels → transmitter synthesis → binding of transmitter to postsynaptic receptor → removal of transmitter
e. Breakdown of calcium channels → transmitter synthesis → binding of transmitter to presynaptic receptor → reuptake of transmitter

**128.** Epileptiform activity is believed to include the activation of

a. AMPA receptors alone
b. Glutamate receptors alone
c. Metabotropic receptors alone
d. Both AMPA and glutamate receptors
e. Both AMPA and metabotropic receptors

**129.** Monoamines differ from neuroactive peptides in which of the following ways?

a. Monoamines are synthesized only in the cell body of neurons
b. Synthesis of monoamines is governed by messenger RNA on ribosomes, which is not true for neuroactive peptides
c. Monoamines are generally synthesized as part of a larger precursor molecule called a prohormone
d. Monoamine neurons are generally regarded as having only excitatory properties, while peptides are inhibitory
e. Monoamine neurons are principally found within brainstem nuclei, while peptide-containing neurons are found throughout the brain

**130.** An enzyme that is directly responsible for the degradation of norepinephrine is

a. Tryptophan hydroxylase
b. Tyrosine hydroxylase
c. Dopamine beta-hydroxylase
d. Catechol-O-methyltransferase
e. Choline acetyltransferase

**131.** Phenylketonuria is a disease that occurs when

a. Ineffective enzyme activity leads to phenylalanine levels that are abnormally high
b. Phenylalanine is converted to tyrosine in excessive amounts, leading to abnormal levels of catecholamines in the brain
c. Tyrosine cannot be converted to DOPA
d. Dopamine cannot be converted to norepinephrine
e. Catecholamine levels remain extremely high as a result of the failure of monoamine oxidase to degrade norepinephrine and dopamine

**132.** A long-lasting depletion of norepinephrine can be produced by administration of

a. Amphetamine
b. Apomorphine
c. Clonidine
d. Reserpine
e. Yohimbine

**133.** In a recent study, it was observed that when catecholamine is released from its terminal endings, further release of this transmitter is temporarily blocked. A similar attenuation of release of catecholamine was noted when an agonist was administered to the experimental preparation. These results are best understood in terms of

a. The presence of a GABAergic neuron at the synapse
b. Postsynaptic inhibition
c. The presence of presynaptic autoreceptors
d. Destruction of the catecholamine cell body
e. Collateral inhibition

**134.** Removal of norephinephrine from the region of the synaptic cleft may be achieved by which of the following mechanisms?

a. Reuptake
b. Enzymatic degradation
c. Diffusion
d. A combination of enzymatic degradation and diffusion
e. A combination of enzymatic degradation, diffusion, and reuptake

# NEUROTRANSMITTERS

## Answers

**90–94. The answers are: 90-d, 91-c, 92-a, 93-e, 94-b.** (*Cooper, 7/e, pp 230–244, 297–301, 353–361. Kandel, 3/e, pp 215–217.*) The biosynthesis of catecholamines includes the following steps: tyrosine (A) is converted into dihydroxyphenylalanine (DOPA) (C) by tyrosine hydroxylase (E). DOPA is then decarboxylated by a decarboxylase to form dopamine (and $CO_2$). The conversion of dopamine to norepinephrine comes about by the action of the enzyme dopamine β-hydroxylase (B). The rate-limiting enzyme in the biosynthesis of serotonin is tryptophan hydroxylase (D). In this process, tryptophan is converted to 5-hydroxytryptophan by tryptophan hydroxylase and by 5-hydroxytryptophan decarboxylase into serotonin.

**95–99. The answers are: 95-d, 96-a, 97-b, 98-h, 99-c.** (*Cooper, 7/e, pp 230–244, 297–301. Kandel, 3/e, pp 215–217.*) In the biosynthesis of catecholamines, the final stage includes the conversion of norepinephrine (D) into epinephrine by the enzyme phenylethanolamine-N-methyltransferase. 5,7-Dihydroxytryptamine (5,7-DHT) is a neurotoxic compound that selectively destroys serotonin (A) neurons. For this reason, it has been widely used in neurochemical and neuropharmacologic studies. Similarly, the drug *p*-chlorophenylalanine (B) depletes serotonin levels in the brain and, thus, has also been widely used in research. Catecholamines may be metabolically degraded by monoamine oxidase (H) or by catechol-*O*-methyltransferase.

**100–104. The answers are: 100-f, 101-i, 102-g, 103-b, 104-D.** (*Cooper, 7/e, pp 162–176, 211–220, 295, 364, 500–501. Kandel, 3/e, pp 162, 213–224, 395–398, 649–656, 683–698.*) Glycine (F) has been identified by electrophysiologic methods as an inhibitory neurotransmitter of spinal interneurons. Other studies have indicated that it may also be an inhibitory transmitter in the retina. Serotonin neurons (I) are localized in clusters of cells along the midline of the brain at the level of the pons and caudal midbrain.

These groups of neurons are referred to as "raphe" neurons and constitute the primary, if not exclusive, source of serotonin that is distributed to both the forebrain and brainstem. The largest afferent source for the neostriatum is the cerebral cortex. The neurotransmitter of this corticostriate projection has now been identified as glutamate (G). The majority of dopamine (B) neurons are located in the ventral tegmental area, interpeduncular nucleus, and pars compacta of the substantia nigra. Fibers from the ventral tegmental area and interpeduncular nucleus supply most of the forebrain, including the cerebral cortex. Dopaminergic neurons from the pars compacta of the substantia nigra supply the neostriatum. Acetylcholine (D) is generally regarded as an excitatory neurotransmitter and is found over wide regions of the central nervous system. Of particular significance is the role of the nucleus basalis of the rostrobasal forebrain, which contains high concentrations of cholinergic neurons that supply the cerebral cortex. Loss of these cholinergic neurons has been implicated in the development of Alzheimer's disease.

**105–109. The answers are: 105-a, 106-e, 107-f, 108-d, 109-g.** (*Cooper, 7/e, pp 126–127, 139–154, 423–426, 436–443. Kandel, 3/e, pp 394–397. Siegel, 5/e, pp 325, 334–335, 347, 393–397.*) Much of the norepinephrine (A) that is distributed throughout the forebrain arises from small groups of nuclei located within the lower brainstem. One such nucleus, which contributes the largest quantities of norepinephrine-containing fibers to the forebrain, is the locus ceruleus. Enkephalin (E) neurons located in the midbrain periaqueductal gray (PAG) are generally considered to be inhibitory neurons. In the PAG, they form the cell bodies for the first link in a descending pathway for the control of ascending nociceptive signals. Substance P (F) is an excitatory neurotransmitter that is found over wide regions of the central nervous system. Within the spinal cord, it has been shown that nociceptive afferent fibers, which terminate in the dorsal horn, contain substance P as a neurotransmitter. Gamma aminobutyric acid (GABA) is an inhibitory neurotransmitter. Direct antagonists for this neurotransmitter (e.g., bicuculline) have been developed. Benzodiazepines potentiate the action of tonically released GABA (D) by displacing an endogenous inhibitor of receptor binding. Benzodiazepines may do this by modifying the affinity of GABA for its own receptor or by coupling the GABA receptor to the chloride ion channel. Within the hypothalamus, there exists a class of releasing factors that significantly influence the synthesis of tropic hormones produced in the pituitary. Moreover, they have properties similar to those of neurotransmitters. One such factor is somatostatin (G), which serves to inhibit the secretion of growth hormone.

**110–114. The answers are: 110-c, 111-g, 112-a, 113-d, 114-e.** (*Cooper, 7/e, pp 261, 325, 329, 342.*) For many of the neurotransmitters that have been studied in recent years, different receptor subtypes have been identified for which specific agonist and antagonist compounds have been developed. The significance of the development of these compounds is that they can be used as experimental tools to determine the physiologic role of different receptors. They have also been used effectively in the treatment of various disorders. For norepinephrine, the following general classes of receptors have been identified: $alpha_1$, $alpha_2$, $beta_1$, and $beta_2$. Prazosin (C) is a selective $alpha_1$-receptor antagonist; clonidine (G) is a selective $alpha_2$-receptor antagonist; yohimbine (A) is a selective $alpha_2$-receptor antagonist; and metoprolol (D) is a selective $beta_1$-adrenergic receptor antagonist. For dopamine, two main classes have been identified. These include dopamine $D_1$ and $D_2$ receptors. Within each group of receptors, recent discoveries have shown that there are several subtypes of receptors that exist (i.e., for $D_1$: $D_1$ and $D_5$ receptors; and for $D_2$: $D_2$, $D_3$, and $D_4$ receptors). Sulpiride (E) is a selective dopamine $D_2$-receptor antagonist.

**115–119. The answers are: 115-h, 116-b, 117-d, 118-e, 119-c.** (*Cooper, 7/e, pp 214–222, 431–438. Siegel, 5/e, pp 304–305, 325–336.*) Recent research over the past two decades has identified a number of different opiate receptors. These include $\mu$, $\delta$, and $\kappa$ receptors. Morphine (H) has been shown to have $\mu$ properties. Dynorphin (C) is a $\kappa$ agonist, and naloxone (B) is a nonspecific antagonist that preferentially acts upon $\mu$ receptors. Two different classes of cholinergic receptors have been identified—muscarinic and nicotinic receptors. Oxotremorine (D) is a selective muscarinic agonist. A wide variety of serotonin receptor subtypes have also been identified. Clozapine (E) is a novel antipsychotic drug that acts as an antagonist at $5\text{-}HT_2$ and $5\text{-}HT_{1C}$ receptor sites.

**120–122. The answers are: 120-b, 121-a, 122-c.** (*Siegel, 5/e, pp 302–303, 310–311, 343–347.*) The hormone melatonin (5-methoxy-*N*-acetyltryptamine) is found in the pineal gland. The pineal gland contains the necessary enzymes to synthesize serotonin (B) from tryptophan as well as to convert serotonin into melatonin. Serotonin is converted by the enzyme serotonin *N*-acetyltransferase to *N*-acetylserotonin and to melatonin by the enzyme 5-hydroxyindole-*O*-

methyltransferase. Immunohistochemical studies have revealed the presence of histamine (A) in cell bodies within the central nervous system. However, these studies have identified such cells only in the tuberomamillary nucleus of the posterior aspect of the hypothalamus. Since this region of the hypothalamus has widespread projections to other parts of the central nervous system, including the ependymal wall of the ventricle, it is quite possible that it participates in a wide variety of functions associated with the hypothalamus as well as with other regions, such as the midbrain periaqueductal gray. Vasopressin (C) is produced mainly from magnocellular neurons of the hypothalamus. The hormone is released into the capillaries of the posterior pituitary. When it is released into the vascular system, it stimulates the kidney to conserve water.

**123–126. The answers are: 123-f, 124-d, 125-c, 126-a.** *(Cooper, 7/e, pp 139–154, 178–190. Siegel, 5/e, pp 368–378.)* With respect to GABA, receptor subtypes include $GABA_A$ and $GABA_B$. Baclofen is a selective $GABA_B$ receptor (F) agonist. AMPA (D) is one of several classes of ionotropic glutamate receptors and functions as a synaptic receptor for fast excitatory synaptic transmission mediated through glutamate. Selective antagonists for AMPA are known. For example, quinoxalinediones, such as 6-nitro-7-sulphamobenzo[f] quinoxaline-2,3-dione (NBQX), function as selective competitive antagonists of AMPA receptors and have little effect upon other receptors. NMDA (C) receptors are unique among receptors in that they require the simultaneous binding of two different agonists for their activation. NMDA ion channels are opened after such compounds as glutamate and glycine are applied to the membranes that include NMDA receptors. Recent evidence has shown that a metabotropic glutamate receptor, L-AP4 (A), is present in the retina. Activation of this receptor may serve to hyperpolarize bipolar neurons within the retina. Glutamate activation (of this receptor) constitutes an unusual action because most neurons in the CNS are depolarized by glutamate.

**127. The answer is b.** *(Kandel, 3/e, pp 213–215.)* Initially, final synthesis of the transmitter takes place in the neuron. The transmitter is then present in the presynaptic terminal and is released into the synaptic cleft where it binds to the postsynaptic receptor. Finally, it is removed from the synaptic cleft or destroyed. Recall also that a necessary stimulus for the release of transmitter is the influx of calcium (through calcium channels) into the synaptic terminal.

**128. The answer is d.** (*Siegel, 5/e, pp 371–372, 380–386.*) Excitatory amino acids and, in particular, the glutamate family of compounds have long been thought to play an important role in epileptiform activity. Epileptiform activity typically includes AMPA receptor activation. However, as the seizure becomes more intense, there is increased involvement of NMDA receptors. This is evidenced by the facts that NMDA antagonists can reduce the intensity and length of the seizure activity and that, following removal of human epileptic hippocampal tissue, there is an upregulation of both AMPA and NMDA receptors. Metabotropic glutamate receptors have been shown to be present in the retina but have not yet been demonstrated to be present in regions of the brain that are typically epileptogenic.

**129. The answer is e.** (*Cooper, 7/e, pp 431–438. Kandel, 3/e, pp 217–221.*) Peptides differ from other neurotransmitters in several ways. Monoamines can be formed in all parts of the neuron with the completion of synthesis in the nerve terminal. In contrast, peptides are formed as a result of messenger RNA that is directed upon ribosomes, thus limiting the site of synthesis to the cell body where the processing is accomplished by the endoplasmic reticulum and Golgi apparatus. Typically, different neuroactive peptides are cleaved from a single, much larger molecule (a prohormone) that has no biologic activity. The active peptide is cleaved by specific peptidases and is ultimately transported down the axon to the nerve terminal. In addition, the overwhelming majority of monoamine neurons are situated in the brainstem, while neuroactive peptides can be found over widespread regions of both the brainstem and forebrain, and, in particular, limbic structures. Both monoamines and peptides may display inhibitory as well as excitatory properties. For example, enkephalins are generally inhibitory, while substance P neurons are excitatory. Monoamine neurons may have excitatory effects in one region of the brain and inhibitory effects in another region.

**130. The answer is d.** (*Cooper, 7/e, pp 196–201, 252, 355. Kandel, 3/e, pp 213–221.*) Tryptophan hydroxylase, tyrosine hydroxylase, and choline acetyltransferase are enzymes that are critical for the biosynthesis of serotonin, catecholamines, and acetylcholine, respectively. Dopamine beta-hydroxylase converts dopamine to norepinephrine. Catechol-*O*-methyltransferase and monoamine oxidase are critical for the metabolic degradation of catecholamines.

**131. The answer is a.** *(Cooper, 7/e, pp 230–231, 482. Kandel, 3/e, p 993.)* Phenylketonuria (PKU) is caused by a deficiency (i.e., structural mutation) in phenylalanine hydroxylase, which has significantly reduced levels of enzyme activity. This defect results in abnormally high levels of phenylalanine with diminished levels of tyrosine. An accumulation of phenylalanine can result in brain damage whose features include mental retardation, seizures, and aggressive tendencies.

**132. The answer is d.** *(Cooper, 6/e, pp 254–258, 284–285.)* Reserpine interferes with the uptake storage mechanism associated with amine granules, which results in destruction of these granules. Administration of this drug will produce longlasting depletion of norepinephrine. Amphetamine blocks the reuptake mechanism and thus produces a net increase in the release of norepinephrine. Apomorphine is a nonspecific dopamine agonist, clonidine is an $alpha_2$-receptor agonist, and yohimbine is an $alpha_2$-receptor antagonist.

**133. The answer is c.** *(Cooper, 7/e, pp 282–285. Kandel, 3/e, pp 207–208.)* These findings can best be explained in terms of a mechanism that involves presynaptic autoreceptors. These receptors modulate the release of a catecholamine by responding to the concentration of this transmitter within the synapse. It thus represents a specific negative feedback mechanism. For example, if the concentration of transmitter in the synapse is high, then release will likely be inhibited. Less inhibition (i.e., more transmitter release) will occur if concentrations are low. Other choices are obviously incorrect. The presence of a GABAergic neuron at the synapse, postsynaptic inhibition, and collateral inhibition are unrelated since they refer to events associated with the postsynaptic neuron, not the catecholamine (presynaptic) neuron. As a result of the phasic nature of this phenomenon, destruction of the catecholamine cell body would produce events that were not phasic; indeed, there would be permanent loss of the neuron's capacity to release transmitter.

**134. The answer is e.** *(Kandel, 3/e, pp 232–233.)* There are three mechanisms by which a transmitter is removed from the region of the synaptic cleft. The most common one is reuptake in which transporter molecules mediate high-affinity reuptake that is specific for the transmitter in question. Other mechanisms include diffusion, which removes some components of the transmitter substance, and enzymatic degradation of the amine achieved by the enzymes monoamine oxidase and catechol-*O*-methyltransferase.

# THE SPINAL CORD

## Questions

**DIRECTIONS:** The questions below consist of lettered headings followed by a set of numbered items. For each numbered item select the **one** heading with which it is **most** closely associated. Each lettered heading may be used **once, more than once, or not at all.**

**Questions 135–140**

Match each description with the appropriate disorder.

a. Amyotrophic lateral sclerosis
b. Hemisection of the spinal cord
c. Multiple sclerosis
d. Neurologic effects of pernicious anemia involving vitamin $B_{12}$ deficiency
e. Syringomyelia
f. Tabes dorsalis
g. Bell's palsy
h. Leukoencephalopathy
i. Nystagmus

**135.** Ipsilateral loss of position sense and contralateral loss of pain and temperature, both below the level of the lesion

**136.** Deficit limited to a 1-2 segmental loss of pain and temperature bilaterally with additional evidence of an ipsilateral lower motor neuron paralysis and Horner's syndrome

**137.** Bilateral loss of position sense and bilateral upper motor neuron paralysis

**138.** Evidence of bilateral upper and lower motor neuron paralysis

**139.** Loss of position and vibratory sense with accompanying ataxia

**140.** Demyelinating disease that affects the white matter of the brain and spinal cord and causes a reduced conduction velocity

## Questions 141–149

Match each description with the appropriate structure on the cross-section of the spinal cord.

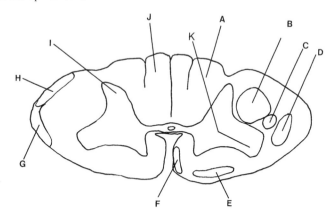

**141.** First-order neurons that transmit sensory information from the upper limbs to the medulla

**142.** Pathway that transmits sensory signals directly to the thalamus

**143.** Fibers that originate from the contralateral cerebral cortex

**144.** Fibers that arise from the midbrain and facilitate flexor motor neurons

**145.** Fibers that facilitate extensor motor neurons

**146.** Second-order neurons that transmit information from muscle spindles to the cerebellum

**147.** Region of spinal cord that receives direct sensory inputs from fibers mediating pain and temperature sensation

**148.** Fibers that arise from the ipsilateral cerebral cortex

**149.** Fibers that reach the cerebellum via the superior cerebellar peduncle

## Questions 150–153

Each effect below may be caused by a lesion at a particular site. Use the previous diagram to locate the site of each causative lesion.

**150.** Lower motor neuron deficit

**151.** Upper motor neuron deficit

**152.** Alleviation of pain associated with the lower limb

**153.** Ataxia of movement

## Questions 154–156

Match each neuron with the appropriate structure.

a. Unmyelinated C fibers
b. Extrafusal muscle fibers
c. Polar region of muscle spindle
d. 1A fibers
e. General visceral efferent fibers
f. High-threshold receptor
g. Special visceral afferent fibers

**154.** Alpha motor neurons

**155.** Gamma motor neurons

**156.** Neurons of intermediolateral cell column

**DIRECTIONS:**    Each question below contains five suggested responses. Select the **one best** response to each question.

**157.** The level of the section of the spinal cord depicted on the previous diagram is

a. Sacral
b. Lower lumbar
c. Upper lumbar
d. Thoracic
e. Cervical

**158.** First-order sensory neurons that terminate in laminas I and II of the spinal cord convey mainly

a. Tactile sensation
b. Pain and temperature sensation
c. Unconscious proprioception limited to inputs from muscle spindles
d. Unconscious proprioception limited to inputs from Golgi tendon organs
e. Inputs associated with pressure receptors

**159.** It has been established that the transmitter released by the axon terminals of first-order pain and temperature fibers is most likely

a. Enkephalins
b. Acetylcholine
c. Substance P
d. Gamma aminobutyric acid (GABA)
e. Serotonin

**160.** Which of the following statements concerning the zone of Lissauer is true?

a. Many fibers that convey unconscious proprioception enter this zone
b. This zone is composed of coarse, heavily myelinated fibers
c. Fibers within the zone of Lissauer may ascend or descend several segments
d. These fibers synapse with alpha motor neurons of extensor muscles
e. Cells in this zone typically project to thalamic nuclei

**161.** Which of the following statements concerning the nucleus dorsalis of Clarke is correct?

a. It is generally regarded as a nucleus associated with autonomic functions
b. It contains second-order neurons for the transmission of unconscious proprioceptive information
c. It contains second-order neurons for the transmission of information from pain receptors
d. Fibers originating from this nucleus cross in the spinal cord
e. This nucleus is found principally at cervical levels of the cord

**162.** Which of the following arrangements best describes the somatotopic organization of the neurons situated in the ventral horn of the spinal cord?

a. Neurons innervating flexor muscles lie ventral to those innervating extensors, and neurons innervating the muscles of the hand lie lateral to those innervating the trunk
b. Neurons innervating flexor muscles lie dorsal to those innervating extensors, and neurons innervating the muscles of the hand lie medial to those innervating the trunk
c. Neurons innervating flexor muscles lie dorsal to those innervating extensors, and neurons innervating the muscles of the hand lie lateral to those innervating the trunk
d. Neurons innervating the muscles of the hand lie lateral to those innervating the trunk, but those innervating flexor and extensor muscles are not topographically segregated
e. Neurons innervating the muscles of the hand lie dorsal to those innervating the trunk, and those innervating flexor muscles lie medial to those innervating extensors

**163.** Which of the following statements correctly characterizes the descending component of the medial longitudinal fasciculus (MLF)?

a. The descending component of the MLF contains fibers arising from the inferior and lateral vestibular nuclei
b. The descending component of the MLF contains fibers that originate in large part in the medial vestibular nucleus and play a role in the regulation of labyrinthine modulation of head position
c. Descending fibers of the MLF are contained within the ventrolateral aspect of the white matter of the spinal cord in a position just lateral to the lateral vestibulospinal and lateral reticulospinal tracts
d. Descending fibers of the MLF suppress extensor reflex activity of the lower limbs of the contralateral side
e. The descending component of the MLF relays impulses from several forebrain nuclei to the intermediolateral cell column of the spinal cord for the regulation of blood pressure

**164.** Which of the following pathways all cross in the spinal cord?

a. Lateral spinothalamic tract, anterior spinothalamic tract, posterior spinocerebellar tract
b. Anterior spinothalamic tract, lateral spinothalamic tract, anterior corticospinal tract
c. Anterior spinocerebellar tract, posterior spinocerebellar tract, lateral vestibulospinal tract
d. Anterior corticospinal tract, lateral spinothalamic tract, dorsal columns
e. Medial vestibulospinal tract, lateral spinothalamic tract, anterior spinothalamic tract

**165.** Which of the following statements concerning muscle spindles is true?

a. They detect the rate of change of muscle length
b. They are high threshold receptors
c. They are arranged in series with the extrafusal muscle fibers
d. They contain a single type of intrafusal fiber
e. They are primarily tension detectors

**166.** The posterior spinocerebellar and anterior spinocerebellar tracts differ in which of the following ways?

a. Fibers from the posterior spinocerebellar tract enter the cerebellum via the superior cerebellar peduncle, while those from the anterior spinocerebellar tract enter the cerebellum via the inferior cerebellar peduncle
b. Fibers of the posterior spinocerebellar tract mediate impulses from the Golgi tendon organs, while those of the anterior spinocerebellar tract mediate impulses arising from the muscle spindles
c. Fibers associated with the posterior spinocerebellar tract signal whole limb movement, while those associated with the anterior spinocerebellar tract signal information concerning the activity of individual muscles
d. Fibers of the posterior spinocerebellar tract arise from all levels of the spinal cord, while those of the anterior spinocerebellar tract arise only from cervical levels
e. The posterior spinocerebellar tract arises mainly from thoracic levels, while the anterior spinocerebellar tract arises mainly from lumbar levels

**167.** An injury to a patient results in a hemisection of the right half of the spinal cord that extends from T8 to T12. It is probable that the patient will experience

a. Loss of pain and temperature sensation from the right leg; loss of conscious proprioception from the left leg; upper motor neuron paralysis of the left leg

b. Loss of pain and temperature sensation from the left leg; loss of conscious proprioception from the right leg; upper motor neuron paralysis of the left leg

c. Loss of pain and temperature sensation from the left arm and leg; loss of conscious proprioception from the right leg and arm; flaccid paralysis of the right leg

d. Loss of pain and temperature sensation from the left leg and loss of conscious proprioception from the right leg; upper motor neuron paralysis of the right leg

e. Bilateral loss of pain and temperature sensation and conscious proprioception, both from the lower half of the body; upper motor neuron paralysis of the left leg and flaccid paralysis of the right leg

# THE SPINAL CORD

## *Answers*

**135–140.The answers are: 135-b, 136-e, 137-d, 138-a, 139-f, 140-c.**
*(Noback, 5/e, pp 174–175. Nolte, 3/e, pp 150–151.)* One of the most striking features of a hemisection of the spinal cord (i.e., Brown-Séquard's syndrome) (B) is the dissociation of loss of pain/temperature with conscious proprioception. On the side ipsilateral to the lesion, there is loss of conscious proprioception since the first-order dorsal column fibers ascend ipsilaterally. In contrast, there is no loss of pain and temperature, ipsilaterally, below the level of the lesion because second-order neurons decussate near their levels of origin and ascend on the contralateral side uninterrupted by the lesion. And, since the pain and temperature fibers decussate, the second-order ascending fibers conveying information from the contralateral side of the body will be disrupted by the lesion. Fibers associated with conscious proprioception on the contralateral side will be left intact since they remain on the side of entry into the cord.

In syringomyelia (E), a development of long cavities in relationship to the central canal frequently extends into the anterior gray horn and region of the intermediolateral cell column. Thus, such a lesion will result in a segmental loss of pain and temperature bilaterally and may also cause some additional disruption of autonomic functions. An example is Horner's syndrome (i.e., ipsilateral constriction of the pupil, dropping of the upper eyelid, vasodilation, and dryness of the skin of the face), which results from damage to the cell bodies of preganglionic sympathetic neurons. In addition, this lesion extends to the anterior horn where it disrupts lower motor neurons, producing a lower motor neuron or flaccid paralysis of the ipsilateral limb.

In combined systems disease (D), there is damage to the dorsal columns with loss of conscious proprioception combined with damage to the corticospinal tracts, which produces an upper motor neuron paralysis. It is caused by a vitamin $B_{12}$ deficiency.

Amyotrophic lateral sclerosis (A) is a degenerative disease that destroys both upper motor neurons (i.e., corticospinal tracts) and lower motor neurons (i.e., ventral horn cells). Thus, this disorder produces signs of both upper and lower motor neuron disturbances.

In tabes dorsalis (F), a CNS form of syphilis, degeneration of the central processes of dorsal root ganglion cells ensues, resulting in demyelination of portions of the dorsal columns. This damage results in loss of position and vibration sensations as well as ataxia because of the loss of position sense.

In multiple sclerosis (C), demyelination of the white matter of the brain and spinal cord leads to a reduction of conduction velocities, which ultimately produces loss of basic functions that require intact neural circuits.

**141–149. The answers are: 141-a, 142-d, 143-b, 144-c, 145-e, 146-h, 147-i, 148-f, 149-g.** (*Noback, 5/e, pp 144, 148, 149. Nolte, 3/e, pp 134–142.*) Sensory fibers that terminate in the medulla are located in the dorsal columns. Fibers mediating conscious proprioception from the upper limb are contained in the fasciculus cuneatus (A). The lateral spinothalamic tract (D) transmits pain and temperature information directly to the thalamus. The lateral corticospinal tract (B) originates in the contralateral cortex and crosses over at the level of the lower medulla. This important pathway mediates control over volitional movements. When these fibers are cut, there is a clear loss of ability to produce volitional movements. The rubrospinal tract (C), situated adjacent to the lateral corticospinal tract, originates from the red nucleus of the midbrain and facilitates the actions of flexor motor neurons. The lateral vestibulospinal tract (E) powerfully facilitates alpha motor neurons of extensor muscles. This tract is located in the ventral funiculus adjacent to the gray matter. The axons of the cells situated in this part of the gray matter (i.e., ventral horn) innervate extensor motor neurons.

The posterior (or dorsal) spinocerebellar tract (H) transmits information from muscle spindles to the cerebellum via the inferior cerebellar peduncle. This tract is located on the lateral aspect of the lateral funiculus of the cord, just above the anterior (or ventral) spinocerebellar tract. Pain and temperature fibers from the periphery terminate directly in the region of the dorsal horn called the substantia gelatinosa (I). A smaller component of the corticospinal tract, the anterior corticospinal tract (F), originates from the cerebral cortex and passes ipsilaterally to the spinal cord. In its ventromedial position, the fibers are ipsilateral to their cortical origin. Just prior to their termination, many of the fibers are distributed to the contralateral side of the cord. The anterior (or ventral) spinocerebellar tract (G) arises from wide regions of the gray matter of the cord. These fibers pass contralaterally to the lateral aspect of the lateral funiculus to reach a position just below the dorsal spinocerebellar tract. These fibers then ascend to the cerebellum via the superior cerebellar peduncle, conveying information from Golgi tendon organs located in the lower limbs.

**150–153. The answers are: 150-k, 151-b, 152-d, 153-j.** (*Noback, 5/e, pp 155–157. Nolte, 3/e, pp 155–157.*) Ventral horn cells (K) constitute the "final common path" for descending motor pathways controlling movement since they directly innervate skeletal muscle. Therefore, they are referred to as "lower motor neurons," and lesions involving any component of these neurons result in a lower motor neuron deficit. The deficit is characterized by a flaccid paralysis of the muscle groups innervated by these neurons. In contrast, neurons from the cerebral cortex (and elsewhere in the brain) that pass in the lateral funiculus of the cord (B) and innervate ventral horn cells rather than skeletal muscle are referred to as "upper motor neurons." Lesions of these fibers produce an upper motor neuron syndrome, which is characterized by a spastic paralysis. The lateral spinothalamic tract (D) conveys pain and temperature signals to the thalamus. Surgical (or other) damage to these fibers will disrupt the transmission of pain signals and alleviate pain from the lower (as well as upper) limbs. The fasciculus gracilis (J) conveys, in part, information from joint capsules to the brain. Disruption of these fibers will block the transmission to the cerebral cortex of these signals that indicate the position of the limb following or preceding movement of that limb. Such loss will prevent the necessary feedback signals concerning one's position in space to reach the cortex. As a result, there will be a compensatory motor response characterized by a wide ataxic gait.

**154–156. The answers are: 154-b, 155-c, 156-e.** (*Kandel, 3/e, pp 569–575, 577, 585–590.*) Alpha motor neurons innervate extrafusal muscle fibers (B) to produce contraction of the muscle and movement of the limb. Gamma motor neurons innervate the polar region of the muscle spindle (C). When activated, these neurons help to reset the position of the muscle spindle and to increase the likelihood that some external stimulus will activate the spindle. The intermediolateral cell column of thoracic, lumbar, and sacral levels contains the cell bodies of preganglionic neurons of the sympathetic and parasympathetic nervous systems, respectively. Accordingly, these fibers are classified as general visceral efferent fibers (E).

**157. The answer is e.** (*Noback, 5/e, p 110. Nolte, 3/e, pp 123–125.*) The cervical level of the spinal cord can be distinguished from other levels of the cord by the following characteristics: the presence of a well-defined fasciculus cuneatus medullae spinalis, situated immediately lateral to the fasciculus gracilis medullae spinalis; the presence of well-defined motor nuclei that are clumped into six different groups, three of which can be distinguished; an absence of an intermediolateral cell column; and relatively extensive quantities of both white and gray matter.

**158. The answer is b.** (*Nolte, 3/e, pp 136–139.*) First-order neurons that convey pain and temperature sensations to the spinal cord terminate principally in laminae I and II upon dendrites of cells located in other laminae. For the most part, tactile and pressure sensations are carried by the dorsal column–medial lemniscal systems, which terminate in the lower medulla. Fibers that mediate unconscious proprioception terminate in the nucleus dorsalis of Clarke.

**159. The answer is c.** (*Noback, 5/e, pp 126–130.*) Immunocytochemical studies have demonstrated that the sensory neurons that terminate in laminae I and II of the dorsal horn of the spinal cord stain intensely for substance P. These neurons are believed to mediate pain impulses. Other transmitter substances, while present within the spinal cord, have not been associated directly with first-order sensory afferent fibers.

**160. The answer is c.** (*Nolte, 3/e, pp 136–140.*) The zone of Lissauer, located on the dorsolateral margin of the dorsal horn of the spinal cord, receives many incoming fibers that are either unmyelinated or finely myelinated. These fibers principally mediate pain and temperature sensations. The fibers contained in this bundle may ascend or descend several segments, serving to integrate different levels of the substantia gelatinosa, which receives these inputs. These fibers are not known to make synaptic contact with motor neurons. Neurons in the substantia gelatinosa do not generally ascend beyond the spinal cord.

**161. The answer is b.** (*Noback, 5/e, pp 140–141.*) The nucleus dorsalis of Clarke is situated in the medial aspect of lamina VII of the cord at thoracic and lumbar levels, but does extend up to C8. It receives first-order inputs from fibers that convey muscle spindle and Golgi tendon organ information. Fibers from the nucleus dorsalis run laterally to form the dorsal spinocerebellar tract on the ipsilateral side, which terminates mainly in the anterior lobe of the cerebellum.

**162. The answer is c.** (*Noback, 5/e, pp 156–157.*) The neurons situated in the ventral horn of the gray matter of the cord are somatotopically organized. This relationship is most clearly seen at cervical levels of the cord. The neurons innervating flexors lie dorsal to those innervating extensors, and the neurons innervating the muscles of the trunk are situated medial to those innervating the hand. These relationships take on added significance when one considers the nature of the descending motor pathways that synapse with these cells. For example, fibers associated mainly with the control of the flexor musculature, such as the corticospinal and rubrospinal tracts, are situated at relatively dorsal levels of the lateral funiculus of the cord. Similarly, fibers associated with the regulation of antigravity muscles (i.e., generally the extensor musculature) are situated in a more ventral position. Thus, the somatotopic organization is maintained throughout the brainstem as well as the spinal cord.

**163. The answer is b.** (*Noback, 5/e, pp 186–189. Nolte, 3/e, pp 143–144.*) This pathway originates, in large measure, in the medial vestibular nucleus, although other regions such as the interstitial nucleus of Cajal of the midbrain, superior colliculus (by virtue of the tectospinal tract), and reticular formation also contribute fibers to this bundle. Fibers from the inferior vestibular nucleus project, instead, to the cerebellum and contribute a few fibers to the ascending component of the MLF; the lateral vestibular nucleus is the origin of the lateral vestibulospinal tract and this cell group also contributes fibers to the ascending component of the MLF. A principal descending component of the MLF arises from the medial vestibular nucleus, and, accordingly, this bundle is sometimes referred to as the *medial vestibulospinal tract.* The overall function of the MLF is to help coordinate changes in position or balance with the position of the head and eyes. The descending fibers of the MLF provide the anatomic substrate by which the inputs from the vestibular apparatus can influence the manner in which the head will be positioned. It accomplishes this by modulating upper cervical neurons that innervate muscles of the neck that control the position of the head. Since the projection is to the cervical cord, it would not likely have any direct effect upon extensor reflex activity of the lower limbs. Likewise, these descending fibers do not affect any structures that would cause alterations in blood pressure.

**164. The answer is b.** *(Noback, 5/e, pp 109–111, 126–127, 131–132, 143–144, 147–153, 156–166.)* Both the lateral and anterior spinothalamic tracts cross over to the contralateral white matter of the cord relatively close to their cell bodies of origin and ascend to the thalamus. Similarly, the ventral spinocerebellar tract crosses over to the contralateral side and ascends as a distinct fiber pathway in the far lateral aspect of the white matter immediately below the position occupied by the dorsal spinocerebellar tract. The anterior corticospinal tract represents approximately 10 percent of the fibers descending from the cortex as corticospinal fibers. These fibers pass ipsilaterally through the brainstem to the spinal cord, reaching the anterior funiculus of the cord. Near the level at which these fibers terminate, most anterior corticospinal fibers cross over in the commissure of the spinal cord to supply the intermediate gray of the ventral horn. Posterior spinocerebellar fibers, which arise from the nucleus dorsalis of Clarke, do not cross in the spinal cord. Instead, they pass laterally from their cell of origin and ascend within the dorsal half of the far lateral aspect of the white matter to the cerebellum. Lateral vestibulospinal fibers arise from the lateral vestibular nucleus and descend ipsilaterally within the ventral funiculus to all levels of the spinal cord, where they terminate upon neurons in the ventral horn. Dorsal column fibers are first-order neurons that arise from the periphery and enter the spinal cord at all levels. They ascend ipsilaterally in the dorsal columns to the level of the dorsal column nuclei of the medulla, where they terminate.

**165. The answer is a.** *(Kandel, 3/e, pp 569–579.)* In contrast to Golgi tendon organs, which detect tension, muscle spindles respond to the rate of change in the length of the muscle and are referred to as *velocity detectors.* They are low-threshold detectors and are connected in parallel with the extrafusal muscle fibers. Stretching the muscle results in an elongation of intrafusal fibers, which stretches the sensory nerve endings in the spindle, producing an increase in the discharge rate. The muscle spindle actually contains three different types of intrafusal fibers: dynamic nuclear bag, static nuclear bag, and nuclear chain fibers, all of which are innervated by a single 1A afferent fiber. Static nuclear bag fibers and nuclear chain fibers are innervated by group II afferent fibers. The various properties of these intrafusal fibers combine in generating the firing patterns of the spindle.

**166. The answer is e.** (*Noback, 5/e, pp 150–151, 186, 255–257. Nolte, 3/e, pp 140–142.*) The posterior spinocerebellar tract carries impulses from both muscle spindles and Golgi tendon organs to the cerebellum via the inferior cerebellar peduncle. The anterior spinocerebellar tract supplies inputs to the cerebellum via the superior cerebellar peduncle. The two tracts differ anatomically since the posterior spinocerebellar tract arises mainly from thoracic levels (C8-L2 or L3), while the anterior spinocerebellar tract arises mainly from lumbar levels. The inputs from the anterior spinocerebellar tract are from the Golgi tendon organ. Thus, these tracts also differ functionally in that the dorsal spinocerebellar tract signals information associated with individual muscles, while the anterior spinocerebellar tract signals information associated with groups of muscles (i.e., whole limb movements).

**167. The answer is d.** (*Noback, 5/e, pp 174–175.*) Hemisection of the right side of the spinal cord that involves segments T8 to T12 will result in contralateral loss of pain and temperature sensation below the level of the lesion and ipsilateral loss of conscious proprioception below the level of the lesion. Thus, this patient will experience loss of pain and temperature in the left leg and loss of conscious proprioception in the right leg. In addition, there will be damage to the descending corticospinal fibers that normally are essential for activation of the lower motor neurons that control muscles of the right leg (i.e., upper motor neuron paralysis of the right leg). However, since the lesion is situated below the entry of sensory fibers as well as the origin of anterior horn cells that innervate the upper limbs, no loss of sensation to the upper limbs will ensue, nor will there be a lower or upper motor neuron paralysis of the upper limbs. The pain and temperature fibers ipsilateral to the site of the lesion are unaffected because the second-order neurons decussate at the approximate level of their cell bodies of origin and ascend on the side contralateral to the lesion, leaving this system intact.

# THE AUTONOMIC
# NERVOUS SYSTEM

## Questions

**DIRECTIONS:** Each question below contains five suggested responses. Select the **one best** response to each question.

**168.** Synaptic transmission in autonomic ganglia is primarily

a. Cholinergic
b. Noradrenergic
c. Serotonergic
d. GABAergic
e. Peptidergic

**169.** Which of the following statements concerning the function of peptides in the autonomic nervous system is true?

a. They are present only at preganglionic axon terminals of the parasympathetic nervous system
b. They are present only at postganglionic axon terminals of the parasympathetic nervous system
c. They are present in sympathetic ganglia where they function primarily as neurotransmitters
d. They are present in sympathetic ganglia where they function primarily as neuromodulators
e. They have not been localized in any of the autonomic ganglia

**170.** The carotid sinus reflex involves

a. Baroreceptor afferent fibers from cranial nerve XI
b. Glossopharyngeal efferent fibers
c. Interneurons within the nucleus ambiguus of the medulla
d. Efferent fibers contained in the intermediate component of the facial nerve
e. Vagal efferent fibers

**171.** Calcium currents present in heart muscle cells are

a. Reduced by norepinephrine acting through beta receptors
b. Increased by norepinephrine acting through beta receptors
c. Increased by acetylcholine acting on muscarinic receptors
d. Increased by acetylcholine acting on nicotinic receptors
e. Increased by serotonin acting on serotonin $1_A$ receptors

**172.** Bladder functions are regulated by which of the following combinations of inputs?

a. Vagal and sacral efferent fibers only
b. Vagal, sacral, and descending fibers from the cerebral cortex
c. Lumbar and sacral efferent fibers only
d. Lumbar, sacral, and descending fibers from the cerebral cortex
e. Lumbar, thoracic, and cervical fibers only

**173.** Synthesis and storage of norepinephrine can be prevented by

a. Guanethidine
b. Reserpine
c. Phenoxybenzamine
d. Hexamethonium
e. Metoprolol

**174.** The hypothalamus and amygdala are able to modulate the output of the autonomic nervous system by virtue of their connections with the

a. Ventrolateral nucleus of the thalamus
b. Nucleus accumbens
c. Solitary nucleus
d. Red nucleus
e. Ventral horn cells at the level of C8-T12 of the spinal cord

# THE AUTONOMIC
# NERVOUS SYSTEM

## *Answers*

**168. The answer is a.** *(Kandel, 3/e, pp 765–767.)* The transmitter released from preganglionic endings of both sympathetic and parasympathetic fibers is acetylcholine. The other transmitters listed are not involved at this synapse. Evidence in support of this view is derived, in part, from studies that demonstrated that drugs that block nicotinic receptors (e.g., hexamethonium, curare) also block the output of these systems.

**169. The answer is d.** *(Kandel, 3/e, pp 768–772.)* Recent studies demonstrate that a wide variety of peptides are found within most sympathetic ganglia. Evidence further suggests that these peptides do not act as transmitters, but instead, serve as neuromodulators. In this manner, the action of peptides in autonomic ganglia is to alter the efficiency of neuronal excitability and the effectiveness of cholinergic transmission at autonomic synapses.

**170. The answer is e.** *(Kandel, 3/e, pp 770–772.)* The carotid sinus reflex involves several neuronal elements. The afferent side of the reflex begins with stretch receptors in the walls of the carotid sinus. These receptors signal "pressure" as a result of stretch of the low-capacitance vessel. This causes an afferent volley of action potentials to pass along the glossopharyngeal nerve into the medulla, where the fibers synapse with neurons in the solitary nucleus. These neurons, in turn, synapse upon neurons in the dorsal motor nucleus of the vagus nerve whose axons innervate the heart. Activation of this reflex results in a decrease in heart rate and force of contraction. As a consequence of the decrease in cardiac output, there is an ensuing decrease in blood pressure as well.

**171. The answer is b.** *(Kandel, 3/e, pp 770–772.)* The calcium current of heart muscle cells is enhanced by the release of norepinephrine that acts on beta adrenergic receptors. This effect is additionally mediated by the modulation of potassium current that serves to keep the action potential of the muscle cells constant. The pacemaker current is also affected by this process since its threshold is decreased as a result of activation of beta receptors (which further involves the second messenger system–cAMP-dependent protein kinase). Lowering the threshold of the pacemaker current serves to increase heart rate. Serotonin is not involved in postsynaptic regulation of the heart. Acetylcholine has an inhibitory effect upon heart muscle by acting through different mechanisms.

**172. The answer is d.** *(Kandel, 3/e, pp 773–775.)* The smooth muscle of the bladder is innervated by postganglionic fibers of the sympathetic nervous system that arise from the inferior mesenteric ganglion. This ganglion, in turn, receives its inputs from T12-L2 of the intermediolateral cell column of the spinal cord. The smooth muscle of the bladder also receives inputs from postganglionic parasympathetic fibers that are innervated by preganglionic fibers arising from S2-S4. The external sphincter of the bladder (striated muscle) is innervated by ventral horn cells from the spinal cord. These ventral horn cells, in turn, receive inputs from supraspinal neurons that arise, in part, from the cerebral cortex. It is these neurons that form a part of the substrate for voluntary control over bladder functions.

**173. The answer is b.** *(Guyton, 2/e, pp 283–284.)* Noradrenergic activity can be blocked by a number of mechanisms. Reserpine, for example, prevents the synthesis and storage of norepinephrine in sympathetic nerve terminals. Guanethidine affects noradrenergic transmission by blocking the release of norepinephrine at the sympathetic endings. Competitive alpha receptor blockers include phenoxybenzamine and phentolamine, whereas metoprolol blocks $beta_1$ receptors. Since acetylcholine is the transmitter at preganglionic synapses of both the parasympathetic and sympathetic nervous systems, hexamethonium is an effective ganglionic blocker at these synapses.

**174. The answer is c.** *(Kandel, 3/e, pp 766–767.)* The solitary nucleus of the medulla plays a significant role in the neural control of autonomic functions because it receives input from several different regions of the brain that regulate such functions. These inputs include fibers that arise from the hypothalamus, central nucleus of amygdala, midbrain periaqueductal gray, and sensory processes (i.e., visceral afferents) of the glossopharyngeal and vagus nerves. The last signal changes in blood pressure and levels of oxygen and carbon dioxide in the blood. The ventrolateral nucleus of the thalamus, red nucleus of the midbrain, and ventral horn cells of the spinal cord are associated with somatomotor rather than autonomic function. The nucleus accumbens is believed to be associated with motivational processes.

# THE BRAINSTEM AND CRANIAL NERVES

## Questions

**DIRECTIONS:** The questions below consist of lettered headings followed by a set of numbered items. For each numbered item select the **one** heading with which it is **most** closely associated. Each lettered heading may be used **once, more than once, or not at all.**

### Questions 175–179

Match each group of nerve cells with its proper classification.

a. Special somatic afferent (SSA)
b. Special visceral afferent (SVA)
c. General somatic afferent (GSA)
d. General visceral afferent (GVA)
e. General visceral efferent (GVE)

**175.** Main sensory nucleus of cranial nerve V

**176.** Otic ganglion

**177.** Nodose (inferior) ganglion (ganglion caudalis nervi vagi)

**178.** Pterygopalatine ganglion

**179.** Geniculate ganglion

### Questions 180–187

Match each group of nerve cells with its proper classification.

a. Special somatic afferent (SSA)
b. Special visceral afferent (SVA)
c. General visceral afferent (GVA)
d. General visceral efferent (GVE)
e. Special visceral efferent (SVE)

**180.** Spiral ganglion

**181.** Scarpa's (vestibular) ganglion

**182.** Superior salivatory nucleus

**183.** Trigeminal motor nucleus

**184.** Edinger-Westphal nucleus of cranial nerve III

**185.** Superior vestibular nucleus

**186.** Optic nerve

**187.** Ciliary ganglion

## Questions 188–191

Match each description with the appropriate structure.

a. Solitary nucleus
b. Dorsal motor nucleus of cranial nerve X
c. Medial vestibular nucleus
d. Carotid sinus
e. Lateral vestibular nucleus

**188.** This structure receives first-order baroreceptor afferents

**189.** The descending fibers of the medial longitudinal fasciculus originate here

**190.** Activation of this structure facilitates responses of extensor motor neurons

**191.** This structure contains baroreceptors

## Questions 192–195

Match each description with the appropriate structure.

a. Solitary nucleus
b. Dorsal motor nucleus of cranial nerve X
c. Inferior ganglion
d. Superior ganglion
e. Otic ganglion

**192.** Origin of axons that innervate the heart

**193.** Locus of cell bodies of neurons that innervate the carotid sinus

**194.** Locus of cell bodies of neurons that innervate the external ear

**195.** Origin of projection to parotid gland

## Questions 196–200

For each dysfunction match the lesion most likely to be responsible.

a. Peripheral lesion limited to the left cranial nerve VI
b. Lesion of the left cranial nerve III
c. Lesion of the left cranial nerve IV
d. Lesion of the right medial longitudinal fasciculus
e. Lesion of the caudal aspect of the dorsomedial pons
f. Lesion of the left cranial nerve V
g. Lesion of the ventromedial medulla

**196.** Inability to move right eye to right side together with inability to smile on right side

**197.** Inability to move left eye medially

**198.** Difficulty in walking down a flight of stairs

**199.** Paresis of right ocular adduction and monocular horizontal nystagmus on left upon attempt to gaze to left

**200.** Inability to gaze to the left with the left eye

## Questions 201–204

Match each description with the appropriate structure.

a. Solitary nucleus
b. Nucleus cuneatus
c. Inferior olivary nucleus
d. Dentate nucleus
e. Spinal tract of cranial nerve V

**201.** Fibers arising from this region directly excite Purkinje cells

**202.** These neurons project to the ventral posteromedial (VPM) nucleus of the thalamus

**203.** Fibers arising from these cells innervate the ventrolateral (VL) nucleus of the thalamus

**204.** This structure transmits taste impulses

## Questions 205–208

Match each description with the appropriate structure.

a. Solitary nucleus
b. Dorsal motor nucleus of cranial nerve X
c. Inferior salivatory nucleus
d. Spinal tract of cranial nerve V
e. Nucleus ambiguus

**205.** Origin of glossopharyngeal fibers that innervate pharyngeal muscles

**206.** Origin of fibers that innervate the otic ganglion

**207.** First-order sensory neuron

**208.** Origin of axons that help to mediate the swallowing reflex

## Questions 209–213

Match each type of cell or fiber with the appropriate site.

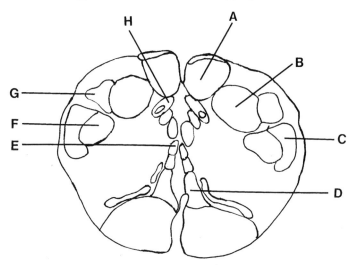

(Adapted from DeArmond, Fig. 41; with permission.)

**209.** Cells in this structure respond to movement of the lower limb

**210.** Cells in this structure respond to a vibratory stimulus applied to the hand

**211.** Fibers in this region mediate reflexes associated with the head

**212.** First-order pain and temperature fibers are found here

**213.** These fibers mediate conscious proprioception and two-point discrimination from the opposite side of the body

## Questions 214–222

Match each description with the appropriate site.

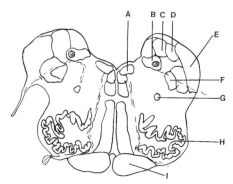

(Adapted from DeArmond, Fig. 44; with permission.)

**214.** This nucleus responds to taste impulses

**215.** Neurons respond to vestibular inputs and project to the spinal cord

**216.** Neurons receive inputs from the red nucleus and spinal cord

**217.** Neurons respond to changes in blood pressure

**218.** Neurons contribute the largest number of fibers that are contained in the inferior cerebellar peduncle

**219.** This nucleus participates in the gag reflex

**220.** Neurons mediate voluntary control of motor functions

**221.** This nucleus innervates muscles of the tongue

**222.** Fibers in this bundle arise from spinal cord and brainstem and project directly to the cerebellum

**Questions 223–228**

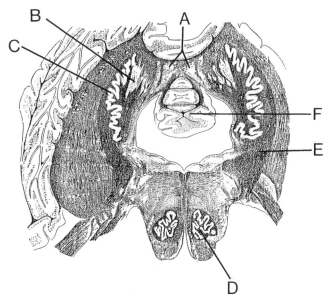

(Adapted from DeArmond, Fig. 14; with permission.)

**223.** Neurons that project to the reticular formation

**224.** Neurons that project to the vestibular nuclei

**225.** Neurons that project to the ventrolateral (VL) nucleus of the thalamus

**226.** Neurons that project primarily to the red nucleus

**227.** Structure that receives inputs from the vermal region of cerebellar cortex

**228.** Neurons that receive inputs from the lateral aspects of the cerebellar hemispheres

## Questions 229–235

Match each description with the correct site.

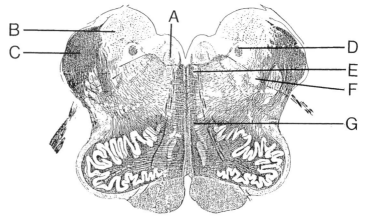

(Adapted from Villiger, Fig. 11; with permission.)

**229.** This structure receives direct inputs from the vestibular apparatus

**230.** These fibers arise from vestibular nuclei

**231.** This structure transmits taste impulses to the thalamus

**232.** This structure is a general somatic efferent (GSE) nucleus

**233.** These fibers arise from dorsal column nuclei

**234.** These fibers transmit pain and temperature signals from the region of the head to the thalamus

**235.** These fibers convey muscle spindle afferents to the cerebellum

## Questions 236–240

Match each structure with the correct site.

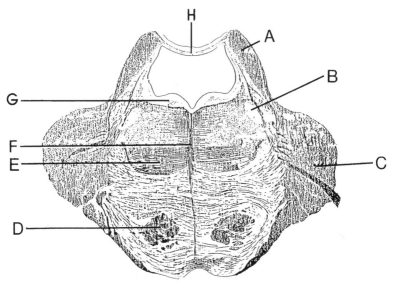

(Adapted from Villiger, Fig. 17; with permission.)

**236.** Axons that are second-order corticocerebellar neurons

**237.** Lower motor neurons

**238.** Upper motor neurons

**239.** Axons that terminate, in part, in the ventrolateral (VL) thalamic nucleus

**240.** Somatotopically organized sensory pathways

## Questions 241–245

Match each structure with the correct site.

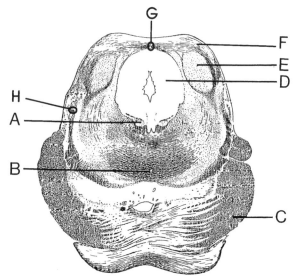

(Adapted from Villiger, Fig. 20; with permission.)

**241.** Sensory relay nucleus

**242.** Fibers that arise from the contralateral dentate and interposed nuclei

**243.** Fibers that arise from the cerebral cortex

**244.** Nucleus that receives inputs from vestibular structures

**245.** Structure that is rich in enkephalin-positive cells and nerve terminals

## Questions 246–250

Match each description with the appropriate site.

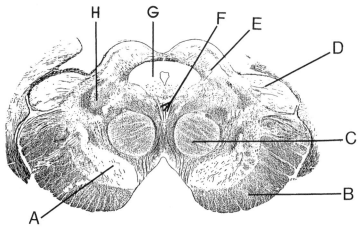

(Adapted from Villiger, Fig. 20; with permission.)

**246.** Site of neurons that respond to moving stimuli

**247.** Specific relay nucleus

**248.** Source of dopaminergic innervation of the striatum

**249.** Nucleus that receives direct inputs from the cerebellum and cerebral cortex

**250.** Lower motor neurons

**DIRECTIONS:**  Each question below contains five suggested responses. Select the **one best** response to each question.

**251.** Which of the following statements concerning the spinal trigeminal nucleus is correct?

a.  It receives direct inputs from first-order descending sensory fibers contained in the ipsilateral spinal tract of cranial nerve V
b.  It projects its axons mainly contralaterally to the ventral posterolateral nucleus of the thalamus
c.  Cells contained in the most caudal aspect of this nucleus respond mainly to mechanical and tactile stimuli
d.  It receives inputs from primary afferent fibers entering the spinal cord at levels C3 and C4
e.  It contains cells whose axons project to the hypothalamus

**252.** Which of the following features concerning the area postrema is true?

a.  It is located in the ventral medulla at a position caudal to the fourth ventricle
b.  It is considered part of the brain because the cells of this structure are protected by the blood-brain barrier
c.  It plays a role in the regulation of emetic functions
d.  Its cells synthesize norepinephrine
e.  It receives major inputs from the forebrain

**253.** The vagus nerve (cranial nerve X) includes which of the following components?

a.  General somatic afferent, special visceral afferent, general visceral afferent, and general visceral efferent
b.  Special visceral afferent, special sensory afferent, general visceral afferent, and general visceral efferent
c.  General visceral afferent and general visceral efferent only
d.  General visceral efferent and special visceral efferent only
e.  Special visceral efferent, general visceral efferent, and general visceral afferent only

**254.** Lesions involving the dorsolateral medulla can produce

a.  Loss of pain and thermal sensation on the contralateral half of the face
b.  Loss of pain and temperature sensation on the ipsilateral side of the body
c.  Dysphonia
d.  Hemiparesis
e.  Intention tremor

**255.** Which of the following statements concerning the olivocochlear bundle is correct?

a. It arises from the inferior olivary nucleus and projects to the cochlea
b. Stimulation of it inhibits acoustic fiber responses to auditory stimuli
c. It communicates directly with the medial lemniscus
d. It can be seen easily in brainstem sections taken from the upper pons
e. It is part of the ascending auditory pathway to the dorsal cochlea nucleus

**256.** Unilateral deafness may result from a lesion of

a. The auditory cortex of one side
b. The lateral lemniscus of one side
c. Cranial nerve VIII on one side
d. The medial geniculate
e. The medial lemniscus

**257.** Which of the following contains first-order sensory neurons with their cell bodies located within the central nervous system?

a. Geniculate ganglion
b. Spiral ganglion
c. Mesencephalic nucleus of cranial nerve V
d. Solitary nucleus
e. Scarpa's ganglia

**258.** In a lateral gaze paralysis, both eyes are conjugatively directed to the side opposite the lesion. In this condition, the locus of the lesion is

a. Root fibers of cranial nerve III
b. Nucleus of cranial nerve III
c. Root fibers of cranial nerve VI
d. Nucleus of cranial nerve VI
e. Nucleus and root fibers of cranial nerve IV

**259.** Which of the following statements concerning the paramedian pontine reticular formation is true?

a. It projects fibers directly to the hypoglossal nucleus
b. Bilateral lesions cause a partial deafness
c. It projects its fibers to the basal ganglia
d. It is a critical site for the integration of impulses regulating vertical and horizontal gaze
e. It is a major site of noradrenergic fibers that project to the forebrain

**260.** A patient displays an ipsilateral paralysis of lateral gaze coupled with a contralateral hemiplegia. A lesion is most likely situated in the

a. Ventromedial medulla
b. Dorsomedial medulla
c. Ventrocaudal pons
d. Dorsorostral pons
e. Ventromedial midbrain

**261.** Which of the following cranial nerves all carry special visceral afferent fibers?

a. V, VII, and IX
b. III, VI, and XII
c. IX, X, and XI
d. II, VII, and VIII
e. I, VII, and IX

**262.** A patient displays the following constellation of symptoms: upper motor neuron paralysis of the left leg, paralysis of the lower half of the left side of the face, and a left homonymous hemianopsia. The lesion is most likely located in the

a. Medulla
b. Basilar pons
c. Pontine tegmentum
d. Midbrain
e. Forebrain

**263.** A man is unable to move his eyes downward. The lesion is most likely situated in the

a. Medulla
b. Basilar aspect of the pons
c. Pontine tegmentum
d. Midbrain
e. Cerebellum

**264.** A patient is capable of displaying pupillary constriction during an accommodation reaction but not in response to a direct light stimulus. The lesion is most likely present in the

a. Optic nerve
b. Ventral cell column of cranial nerve III
c. Pretectal area
d. Visual cortex
e. Edinger-Westphal nucleus of cranial nerve III

**265.** Structures associated with the taste pathway include the

a. Geniculate ganglion, chorda tympani, and medial lemniscus
b. Solitary nucleus, parabrachial nucleus, and ventral posteromedial nucleus
c. Solitary nucleus, ventral posterolateral nucleus, and postcentral gyrus
d. Solitary nucleus, ventral posteromedial nucleus, and superior parietal lobule
e. Geniculate ganglion and ventral posterolateral nucleus

**Questions 266–269**

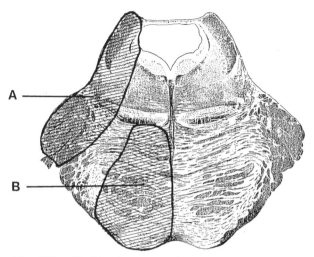

(Adapted from Villiger, Fig. 18; with permission.)

**266.** The lesion at A most likely resulted from an occlusion of the

a. Basilar artery
b. Superior cerebellar artery
c. Anterior spinal artery
d. Vertebral artery
e. Posterior inferior cerebellar artery

**267.** The lesion at B is most likely the result of an occlusion of the

a. Paramedian branch of the basilar artery
b. Circumferential branch of the basilar artery
c. Superior cerebellar artery
d. Anterior inferior cerebellar artery
e. Anterior spinal artery

**268.** Structures affected by the lesion at B include

a. Medial lemniscus
b. Lateral lemniscus
c. Corticospinal tract
d. Medial longitudinal fasciculus
e. Tectospinal tract

**269.** The lesion at B would most likely result in which of the following deficits?

a. Paralysis of the contralateral limbs
b. Loss of conscious proprioception of the contralateral side of the body
c. Nystagmus
d. Lateral gaze paralysis
e. Facial paralysis

**Questions 270–272**

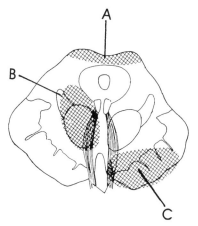

Adapted from Kandel, Fig. 46 l 4; with permission.)

**270.** A patient with the lesion at A will generally show which of the following deficits?

a. Partial blindness
b. Loss of ability to gaze medially
c. Loss of ability to show tracking movements
d. Loss of accommodation reflex
e. Nystagmus

**271.** Which of the following deficits is likely to occur as a result of the lesion at B?

a. Contralateral loss of conscious proprioception
b. Transient tremor of the ipsilateral limb
c. Ipsilateral fourth nerve palsy
d. Hearing loss
e. Contralateral loss of taste sensation

**272.** The deficits associated with the lesion at C are the result of damage to the

a. Substantia nigra and crus cerebri
b. Red nucleus and crus cerebri
c. Crus cerebri and cranial nerve III
d. Red nucleus and substantia nigra
e. Substantia nigra and cranial nerve III

**273.** Which of the following statements best describes the regions of the ventral tegmental area and pars compacta of the substantia nigra?

a. Both regions contain dopaminergic neurons but project to different populations of forebrain structures
b. Both regions provide converging dopaminergic inputs to the hypothalamus
c. Both regions provide converging dopaminergic inputs to the neostriatum
d. Both regions are innervated by GABAergic fibers and project to the cerebral cortex
e. Lesions of either region result in the development of a Parkinsonian-like syndrome

**274.** The principal ascending auditory pathway of the brainstem is the

a. Medial lemniscus
b. Lateral lemniscus
c. Trapezoid body
d. Trigeminal lemniscus
e. Brachium of the superior colliculus

# THE BRAINSTEM AND CRANIAL NERVES

## *Answers*

**175–179. The answers are: 175-c, 176-e, 177-d, 178-e, 179-b.** *(Wilson-Pauwels, pp vii, 50–55, 63, 114–120.)* The mesencephalic nucleus of cranial nerve V receives inputs from the head region associated with unconscious proprioception (i.e., general somatic afferent) (C). The otic ganglion contains postganglionic parasympathetic neurons (in association with cranial nerve IX) that innervate the parotid gland and is therefore classified as a general visceral efferent (E). The nodose ganglion contains the cell bodies of first-order neurons of cranial nerves IX and X, which mediate inputs from visceral organs associated with chemoreceptors and baroreceptors. Accordingly, these neurons are classified as general visceral afferents (D). The pterygopalatine ganglion contains cells whose axons constitute postganglionic fibers for cranial nerve VII that innervate the lacrimal, nasal, and palatine glands. Thus, these fibers are classified as general visceral efferents (E). The geniculate ganglion contains the first-order cell bodies associated with fibers of cranial nerve VII that mediate taste (special visceral afferent) (B) information to the solitary nucleus of the brainstem.

**180–187. The answers are: 180-a, 181-a, 182-d, 183-e, 184-d, 185-a, 186-a, 187-d.** *(Wilson-Pauwels, pp viii, 10–18, 26–39, 50–56, 82–86, 98–106.)* The spiral ganglion and Scarpa's (vestibular) ganglion contain the cell bodies of first-order auditory and vestibular fibers, respectively, that pass to the lower brainstem. These neurons are classified as special somatic afferents (A). The superior salivatory nucleus contains preganglionic parasympathetic neurons for cranial nerve VII that make synaptic contact with neurons in the pterygopalatine and submandibular ganglia and are thus classified as general visceral efferents (D). The motor nucleus of cranial nerve V innervates the muscles of mastication and, since it is derived from the first branchial arch, it is classified as a special visceral efferent nerve (E).

The Edinger-Westphal nucleus of cranial nerve III projects its axons to the ciliary ganglion, whose fibers in turn innervate the ciliary muscles (activation induces the lens to bulge for accommodation), or to the pupillary constrictor muscles for pupillary constriction. Since these are both smooth muscles, the Edinger-Westphal cells constitute preganglionic parasympathetic neurons and the ciliary ganglion cells are postganglionic parasympathetic neurons. Each is classified as a general visceral efferent (D). The superior vestibular nucleus receives direct inputs from first-order vestibular neurons and the optic nerve contains fibers whose origin is the retinal ganglion cells. Accordingly, both of these structures are classified as special somatic afferents (A).

**188–191. The answers are: 188-a, 189-c, 190-e, 191-d.** *(Noback, 5/e, pp 178, 197–200. Wilson-Pauwels, pp viii, 97–136.)* The solitary nucleus (A) receives first-order baroreceptor afferents from cranial nerves IX and X. The descending tract of the medial longitudinal fasciculus (MLF) arises from the medial vestibular nucleus (C). Stimulation of the lateral vestibular nucleus (E) facilitates the responses of extensor motor neurons. Baroreceptors are specialized receptors found in specific regions along the walls of several major blood vessels that respond to increases in blood pressure. In particular, the carotid sinus (D), located at the bifurcation of the common carotid artery, responds to such changes in blood pressure by sending a signal into the central nervous system. The afferent limb of this pathway constitutes a component of a reflex mechanism governing a homeostatic mechanism for the regulation of blood pressure.

**192–195. The answers are: 192-b, 193-c, 194-d, 195-e.** *(Wilson-Pauwels, pp 114–137.)* The dorsal motor nucleus of the vagus nerve (B), located in the dorsal aspect of the lower medulla, gives rise to preganglionic parasympathetic fibers that compose the descending vagus and cause slowing of heart rate upon stimulation. Baroreceptors are located in the carotid sinus and have their cell bodies situated in the inferior ganglion (C) of cranial nerve IX. The external ear is innervated by general somatic afferent fibers of cranial nerve IX whose cell bodies are located in the superior ganglion (D). Axons of cells located in the otic ganglion (E) constitute postganglionic parasympathetic neurons that innervate the parotid gland for controlling salivation.

**196–200. The answers are: 196-e, 197-b, 198-c, 199-d, 200-a.** *(Noback, 5/e, pp 179–197.)* A lesion situated in the caudal aspect of the right dorsomedial pons (E) will affect the nucleus of cranial nerve VI along with surrounding tissue. This will invariably include the fibers of cranial nerve VII, which wrap around the nucleus of cranial nerve VI. As a result, there will be a loss of facial expression on the right side because cranial nerve VII innervates the muscles of facial expression, along with an inability to move the right eye laterally because cranial nerve VI innervates the lateral rectus muscle.

Cranial nerve III innervates all the rectus muscles except the lateral rectus. Therefore, a patient sustaining a lesion of this nerve will not be able to move the eye on the affected side medially (B).

The fourth cranial nerve (C) innervates the superior oblique muscle, which moves the eye downward from a medial position. This movement most often occurs when one walks down a flight of stairs.

A lesion of the right medial longitudinal fasciculus (D) will disrupt axons that arise from the nucleus of cranial nerve VI of the left side that cross over and ascend to the oculomotor complex. Thus, this lesion would produce a dissociation of horizontal eye movements in which gazing to the left would result in a paresis of right ocular adduction together with monocular horizontal nystagmus in the left (abducting) eye.

**201–204.** The answers are: 201-c, 202-a, 203-d, 204-a. (*Noback, 5/e, pp 211, 254–259.*) Climbing fibers arising from the inferior olivary nucleus (C) make synaptic contact with dendrites of Purkinje cells. Stimulation of the inferior olivary nucleus directly excites Purkinje cells, causing these cells to discharge. While several groups of cells within the solitary nuclear complex (A) participate in cardiovascular functions, others serve as a principal relay for the taste system. One of the primary target structures of this nucleus with respect to the taste pathway is the ventral posteromedial (VPM) nucleus of the thalamus. Fibers from the VPM nucleus are then relayed directly to the head region of the postcentral gyrus, which includes cells responsive to neural signals mediating taste information. The efferent pathways of the cerebellum arise from several nuclear groups. One such nucleus is the dentate nucleus (D). Neurons from this structure supply the ventrolateral (VL) nucleus of the thalamus. This projection allows the cerebellum to communicate with the motor cortex since the VL nucleus projects directly to the precentral (primary motor) cortex.

**205–208.** The answers are: 205-e, 206-c, 207-d, 208-e. (*Wilson-Pauwels, pp viii, 60–69, 114–134.*) The nucleus ambiguus (E) gives rise to lower motor neurons of cranial nerve IX. Fibers associated with cranial nerve IX innervate pharyngeal muscles. The nucleus ambiguus also gives rise to axons that compose part of cranial nerve X and innervate laryngeal muscles. Preganglionic parasympathetic neurons of cranial nerve IX arise from the inferior salivatory nucleus (C) and make synapse in the otic ganglion. Surgical destruction of the descending tract of cranial nerve V (D) has been used to eliminate facial pain.

**209–213. The answers are: 209-a, 210-b, 211-e, 212-c, 213-d.** (*Noback, 5/e, pp 143–150, 163–164.*) The nucleus gracilis (A) contains cells that respond to movement of the lower limb as a result of joint capsule activation. The nucleus cuneatus (B) contains cells that respond to a variety of stimuli applied to the upper limb, including vibratory stimuli. One component of the descending medial longitudinal fasciculus (MLF) (E) contains fibers that arise from the medial vestibular nucleus that project to cervical levels and contribute to reflex activity associated with the position of the head. Fibers of the medial lemniscus (D) arise from the contralateral dorsal column nuclei and ascend to the ventral posterolateral nucleus (VPL) of the thalamus. These fibers transmit the same information noted above for the dorsal column nuclei, which includes two-point discrimination and conscious proprioception from the opposite side of the body.

**214–222. The answers are: 214-b, 215-c, 216-h, 217-b, 218-h, 219-g, 220-i, 221-a, 222-e.** (*Noback, 5/e, pp 164, 211–214, 254–255. Nolte, 3/e, pp 154–168.*) Different groups of neurons of the solitary complex (B) respond to taste stimuli and to inputs that signal sudden changes in blood pressure. The medial vestibular nucleus (C) receives direct vestibular inputs from the otolith organ and semicircular canals. Axons of medial vestibular neurons descend to the spinal cord in the medial longitudinal fasciculus (MLF) and serve to regulate reflexes associated with the head. The inferior vestibular nucleus (D) also receives vestibular inputs, but does not project its axons to the spinal cord. The inferior olivary nucleus (H) receives inputs from the red nucleus and spinal cord, and it projects its axons through the inferior cerebellar peduncle (where it constitutes its largest component) to the contralateral cerebellar cortex, where they synapse with the dendrites of Purkinje cells.

The nucleus ambiguus (G) is a special visceral efferent (SVE) nucleus that is situated in a position ventrolateral to that of the hypoglossal nucleus. Its axons innervate the muscles of the larynx and pharynx and therefore are essential for the occurrence of such responses as the gag reflex. The pyramids (I), located on the ventromedial aspect of the brainstem, contain fibers that arise from sensorimotor cortex. These neurons serve as essential upper motor neurons that mediate voluntary control of motor functions. The hypoglossal nucleus (A), a general somatic efferent (GSE) nucleus, is located in the dorsomedial aspect of the medulla. Its axons innervate the muscles of the tongue and cause extrusion of the tongue toward the opposite side. Fibers contained in the inferior cerebellar peduncle (E) arise from cells located in both the spinal cord and brainstem.

**223–228.** The answers are: 223-a, 224-a, 225-c, 226-b, 227-a, 228-c. (*Noback, 5/e, pp 255–259. Nolte, 3/e, pp 350–354.*) The efferent projections of the cerebellum arise from three distinct groups of nuclei called deep cerebellar nuclei. The nucleus located in the most medial position is the fastigial nucleus (A). It gives rise to at least two important projections—one that is distributed to the reticular formation and another that is distributed to the vestibular nuclei. The nucleus situated most laterally is the dentate nucleus (C). It projects through the superior cerebellar peduncle and its axons innervate principally the ventrolateral (VL) nucleus of the thalamus. Neurons of the emboliform (B) and globose (not labeled) nuclei lie in an intermediate position between the fastigial and dentate nuclei and are therefore often referred to as the *interposed nuclei*. Their axons project through the superior cerebellar peduncle principally to the red nucleus. The projections from the cerebellar cortex to the deep cerebellar nuclei are topographically organized. Cells located in the far medial aspect of the cerebellar cortex, the vermal region, project (via Purkinje cell axons) to the fastigial nucleus (A). In contrast, the lateral aspects of the cerebellar hemispheres project to the dentate nucleus (C), which is the most lateral of the deep cerebellar nuclei.

**229–235.** The answers are: 229-b, 230-e, 231-d, 232-a, 233-g, 234-f, 235-c. (*Nolte, 3/e, pp 135, 140–142, 155–170, 176–198.*) The inferior vestibular nucleus (B) lies immediately medial to the inferior cerebellar peduncle (shown at C) and receives direct inputs from first-order vestibular fibers that arise from the vestibular apparatus. The medial longitudinal fasciculus (E) contains second-order vestibular fibers, the majority of which ascend in the brainstem to innervate cranial nerve nuclei III, IV, and VI. A small component of this bundle also descends to cervical levels of the spinal cord from the medial vestibular nucleus. The solitary nucleus (D) receives inputs from first-order taste fibers and is thus a special visceral afferent (SVA) nucleus that transmits taste signals to the ventral posteromedial (VPM) nucleus of the thalamus. The solitary nucleus also receives cardiovascular inputs from cranial nerve IX and, for this reason, has properties of a general visceral afferent (GVA) nucleus as well. The hypoglossal nucleus (A) innervates the muscles of the tongue. It is classified as a general somatic efferent (GSE) nucleus because it is derived from somites rather than branchial arches and innervates skeletal muscle.

The medial lemniscus (G) ascends to the thalamus and transmits information associated with conscious proprioception. This bundle constitutes a second-order neuron that arises from the dorsal column nuclei of the lower medulla. The dorsal column nuclei receive first-order signals that mediate conscious proprioception from fibers contained within the dorsal columns of the spinal cord. The spinal nucleus of cranial nerve V (F) receives pain and temperature fibers from first-order trigeminal neurons that arise from the head. The inferior cerebellar peduncle (C) is one of two principal cerebellar afferent pathways. One major fiber group contained within the inferior cerebellar peduncle arises from brainstem structures such as the contralateral inferior olivary nucleus and reticular formation. The other groups of fibers contained within this bundle arise from the spinal cord. Of the fibers that ascend in this bundle from the spinal cord, many constitute second-order muscle spindle afferents that arise from the nucleus dorsalis of Clarke.

**236–240. The answers are: 236-c, 237-b, 238-d, 239-a, 240-e.** (*Nolte, 3/e, pp 134–136, 140–142, 346–350.*) The middle cerebellar peduncle (C) serves as a relay nucleus for the transmission of information from the cerebral cortex to the cerebellum. Fibers in this peduncle arise from the contralateral deep pontine nucleus, which receives its principal afferents from the cerebral cortex. The motor nucleus of cranial nerve V (B) is a lower motor neuron (special visceral efferent) because it innervates the muscles of mastication. Corticobulbar and corticospinal fibers (D) are situated in the ventral aspect of the basilar pons. Fibers of the superior cerebellar peduncle (A) project to both the red nucleus and ventrolateral (VL) nucleus of the thalamus. The medial lemniscus (E) is a somatotopically organized pathway that arises from the dorsal column nuclei and projects to the ventral posterolateral (VPL) nucleus of the thalamus. Fibers of this pathway that arise from the nucleus gracilis (associated with the leg) project to more dorsolateral aspects of the VPL nucleus. Fibers arising from the nucleus cuneatus (associated with the arm) project to more ventromedial aspects of the VPL nucleus.

**241–245. The answers are: 241-e, 242-b, 243-c, 244-a, 245-d.** (*Nolte, 3/e, pp 165–167.*) The inferior colliculus (E) is situated in the caudal aspect of the tectum and is an important relay nucleus for the transmission of auditory information to the cortex from lower levels of the brainstem. The decussation of the superior cerebellar peduncle (B) is also present at caudal levels of the midbrain and is usually seen together with the inferior colliculus. These crossing fibers arise from the dentate and interposed nuclei and terminate in the contralateral red nucleus and ventrolateral (VL) nucleus of the thalamus. The crus cerebri (C) contains fibers that arise from all regions of the cortex and project to all the levels of the brainstem and the spinal cord. The trochlear nucleus (cranial nerve IV) (A), which is situated just below the periaqueductal gray at the level of the inferior colliculus, receives direct inputs from ascending fibers of the medial longitudinal fasciculus that arise from vestibular nuclei. The midbrain periaqueductal gray (D) contains dense quantities of enkephalin-positive cells and nerve terminals. The transmitter (or neuromodulator) enkephalin plays an important role in the regulation of pain and emotional behavior.

**246–250. The answers are: 246-e, 247-d, 248-a, 249-c, 250-f.** (*Nolte, 3/e, pp 165–167.*) The superior colliculus (E), situated at a more rostral level of the tectum, plays an important role in tracking or pursuit of moving stimuli. The medial geniculate nucleus (D), which is part of the forebrain, actually sits over the lateral aspect of the midbrain and can be seen at rostral levels of the midbrain. It is part of an auditory relay system and receives its inputs from the inferior colliculus via fibers of the brachium of the inferior colliculus. The pars compacta is situated in the medial aspect of the substantia nigra (A) and contains dopamine neurons whose axons innervate the striatum. The red nucleus (C), a structure associated with motor functions, receives direct inputs from both the cerebral cortex and the cerebellum. The oculomotor nerve (cranial nerve III) (F), located at the level of the superior colliculus, contains general somatic efferent (GSE) components that innervate extraocular eye muscles and general visceral efferent (GVE) components whose postganglionic fibers innervate smooth muscles associated with pupillary constriction and bulging of the lens.

**251. The answer is a.** *(Nolte, 3/e, pp 187–192.)* The spinal trigeminal nucleus receives its sensory inputs from first-order neurons contained in the ipsilateral descending tract of cranial nerve V. A central property of the spinal trigeminal nucleus is that it is uniquely associated with pain inputs (to the exclusion of the main sensory nucleus and mesencephalic nucleus). Fibers from this nucleus mainly project contralaterally to the ventral posteromedial (VPM) nucleus of the thalamus.

**252. The answer is c.** *(Kandel, 3/e, pp 1055–1056. Nolte, 3/e, p 89.)* The area postrema is of interest because it is a circumventricular organ associated with emetic functions. As a circumventricular organ, the area postrema constitutes a part of the ependymal lining of the brain's ventricular system (in this case, the fourth ventricle). The area postrema contains both fenestrated and non-fenestrated capillaries that allow for enhanced transport, which possibly accounts for the fact that it lies outside the blood-brain barrier. Axons and dendrites from neighboring structures (but not from the forebrain) innervate this structure, which is composed of astroblast-like cells, arterioles, sinusoids, and some neurons. Various peptides (but not monoamine-containing neurons) have also been shown to be present in this structure. Experimental evidence has strongly implicated the area postrema as a chemoreceptor trigger zone for emesis. It responds to digitalis glycosides and apomorphine.

**253. The answer is a.** *(Wilson-Pauwels, pp 126–137.)* Cranial nerve X is a highly complex nerve. It contains a few general somatic afferents from the back of the ear that enter the brain as cranial nerve X but terminate in the trigeminal complex. Special visceral afferents include fibers from chemoreceptors for taste associated with the epiglottis and chemoreceptors in the aortic bodies that sense changes in $O_2$-$CO_2$ levels in the blood. General visceral afferent fibers arise from the trachea, pharynx, larynx, and esophagus and signal changes in blood pressure to the brainstem. Special visceral efferent fibers innervate the constrictor muscles of the pharynx and the intrinsic muscles of the larynx. General visceral efferent fibers constitute part of the cranial aspect of the parasympathetic nervous system; thus, they are preganglionic parasympathetic fibers that innervate the heart, lung, esophagus, and stomach.

**254. The answer is c.** *(Nolte, 3/e, pp 171–174.)* A primary characteristic of a lesion of the dorsolateral medulla is loss of pain and temperature sensation on the contralateral side of the body and ipsilateral half of the face. Damage to the descending tract of the trigeminal nerve and to the spinal nucleus of cranial nerve V will produce loss of sensation on the ipsilateral side of the face. There also will be damage to the lateral spinothalamic tract, which has already crossed at the level of the spinal cord and which conveys pain and temperature sensation from the contralateral side of the body. In addition, fibers arising from the nucleus ambiguus exit laterally from the medulla, and these fibers, which innervate the larynx and pharynx, would also be affected, causing dysphonia. Hemiparesis would not result from this lesion since the pyramidal tract would remain intact. The cerebellum would also be spared and intention tremor associated with cerebellar damage would not occur.

**255. The answer is b.** *(Nolte, 3/e, pp 211–218.)* The olivocochlear bundle is a most interesting pathway because it arises from the region immediately dorsal to the superior olivary nucleus and projects contralaterally back to the hair cells of the cochlea. Stimulation of this bundle results in inhibition or reduction of responses to auditory signals by auditory nerve fibers. There is no evidence that the olivocochlear bundle bears any anatomic or functional relationship to the medial lemniscus. Since the pathway arises from the superior olivary nucleus, which is present at the level of the lower pons, it would not be visible in a section taken from the upper pons.

**256. The answer is c.** *(Nolte, 3/e, pp 211–218.)* Since the auditory relay system is a highly complex pathway in which auditory signals are bilaterally represented at all levels beyond the receptor level, lesions at these levels would not produce a solely unilateral deafness. That could only result when the lesion involves either the receptor or the first-order neurons of the nerve (i.e., cranial nerve VIII itself). The medial lemniscus is not related to the auditory system.

**257. The answer is c.** *(Nolte, 3/e, pp 187–193.)* In general, first-order sensory neurons form ganglia outside the central nervous system. There is one exception—the mesencephalic nucleus of cranial nerve V, which transmits unconscious proprioception (i.e., muscle spindle activity) from jaw muscles. These inputs serve as the first-order neurons for a disynaptic pathway to the cerebellum as well as for a monosynaptic pathway with the motor nucleus of cranial nerve V for the jawclosing reflex.

**258. The answer is d.** *(Nolte, 3/e, pp 182–185.)* Conjugate lateral gaze requires the simultaneous contractions of the lateral rectus muscle of one eye and the medial rectus of the other eye. Recent studies have indicated that there is a region that integrates and coordinates such movements and that the site is part of the nucleus of cranial nerve VI. It is likely that it accomplishes this phenomenon, in part, because ascending axons from the abducens nucleus pass through the medial longitudinal fasciculus to the contralateral nuclei of cranial nerve III. Thus, the abducens nucleus serves not only to innervate the lateral rectus muscle but also to integrate signals necessary for conjugate deviation of the eyes. The abducens nucleus appears to be the only cranial nerve structure where lesions of the root fibers and nucleus fail to display identical effects.

**259. The answer is d.** (*Nolte, 3/e, pp 238–241, 274–277.*) The paramedian pontine reticular formation is an important integrating structure controlling the position of the eyes. It receives inputs from the cerebral cortex (presumably the region of the frontal eye fields) and fibers from the cerebellum, spinal cord, and vestibular complex. Its efferent fibers project to the cerebellum, vestibular complex, pretectal region, interstitial nucleus of Cajal, and nucleus of Darkshevich of the rostral midbrain. These all are nuclei concerned with the regulation of eye position and movements. It is not related to any other known motor or auditory functions, nor has it been shown to contain ascending noradrenergic neurons.

**260. The answer is c.** (*Noback, 5/e, p 247. Nolte, 3/e, pp 182–185.*) In order for a lesion to produce both an ipsilateral gaze paralysis and contralateral hemiplegia, it must be situated in a location where fibers regulating both lateral gaze and movements of the contralateral limbs lie close to each other. The only such location is the ventrocaudal aspect of the pons, where fibers of cranial nerve VI descend toward the ventral surface of the brainstem and where corticospinal fibers are descending toward the spinal cord. The other regions listed in the question do not meet this condition.

**261. The answer is e.** (*Wilson-Pauwels, p viii.*) The group called special visceral afferent fibers is limited to those cranial nerves that convey impulses to the brain associated with olfaction (I) and taste (VII, IX, and X). Since olfaction and taste involve chemical senses, some authors also include cranial nerves IX and X in the group because these nerves contain components involved in signaling changes in $O_2$ and $CO_2$ levels in the blood.

**262. The answer is e.** *(Nolte, 3/e, pp 246–264.)* Because the deficit includes a homonymous hemianopsia, the lesion has to be located somewhere in the forebrain, such as in the region that includes the optic tract and internal capsule on the right side of the brain. The motor neurons of cranial nerve VII as well as spinal cord motor neurons receive cortical fibers that are crossed, which accounts for the fact that motor dysfunctions of the lower face and body involve lesions on the same side.

**263. The answer is d.** *(Wilson-Pauwels, pp 26–47.)* Inability to move the eyes to a downward position may result from a lesion of cranial nerve IV (when the eye is positioned medially) or cranial nerve III (when the eye is positioned laterally). In either case, the cell bodies of origin of these cranial nerves are located in the midbrain.

**264. The answer is c.** *(Nolte, 3/e, pp 300–301.)* This disorder is referred to as the Argyll Robertson pupil and occurs with central nervous system syphilis (tertiary). Although the precise site of the lesion has never been fully established, it is believed to be in the pretectal area. The reasoning is as follows: In the pupillary light reflex, many optic fibers terminate in the pretectal area and superior colliculus region and are then relayed to the autonomic nuclei of cranial nerve III. Impulses from this component of cranial nerve III then synapse with postganglionic parasympathetics that innervate the pupillary constrictor muscles, thus producing pupillary constriction. In the case of the accommodation reflex, retinal impulses first reach the cortex and are then relayed through corticofugal fibers to the brainstem. Some of these fibers are then relayed directly or indirectly to both motor and autonomic components of cranial nerve III, thus activating the muscles required for the accommodation reaction to occur, which includes pupillary constriction.

**265. The answer is b.** *(Kandel, 3/e, pp 524–525. Nolte, 3/e, pp 193–196.)* The solitary nucleus receives first-order neurons from the taste system and thus serves as a critical relay nucleus for the taste pathway. Axons arising from the solitary nucleus project to the ventral posteromedial nucleus of the thalamus and may also synapse in the parabrachial nuclei of the upper pons. Structures such as the ventral posterolateral nucleus, medial lemniscus, and superior parietal lobule are not associated with the taste pathway.

**266. The answer is b.** *(Nolte, 3/e, pp 162–173.)* The superior cerebellar artery supplies the dorsolateral aspect of the upper pons. The basilar artery supplies the medial aspect of the pons. The other arteries (vertebral, anterior spinal, and posterior inferior cerebellar) supply different parts of the medulla. The lateral aspect of the upper pons contains spinothalamic fibers, the lateral lemniscus, and the locus ceruleus (situated just dorsal to the motor nucleus of cranial nerve V which is also affected by the lesion). This lateral pontine lesion produces a syndrome that includes (1) loss of pain and temperature sensation from the contralateral side of the body (damage to the lateral spinothalamic tract), (2) ipsilateral loss of masticatory reflexes (damage to the motor nucleus of cranial nerve V), (3) diminution of hearing (disruption of secondary auditory pathways), and (4) Horner's syndrome (disruption of descending fibers from the hypothalamus and midbrain that mediate autonomic functions).

**267. The answer is a.** *(Kandel, 3/e, pp 726–728.)* The paramedial branch of the basilar artery supplies the ventromedial pons (i.e., medial basilar pons). The circumferential branch supplies more lateral regions of the pons as does the superior cerebellar artery. The anterior spinal and anterior inferior cerebellar arteries supply different parts of the medulla.

**268. The answer is c.** *(Kandel, 3/e, pp 726–728.)* The lesion is restricted to the basilar pons. Thus, the only structure affected by this lesion among the choices given is the corticospinal tract. The other structures listed are situated in the tegmentum of the pons.

**269. The answer is a.** *(Kandel, 3/e, pp 726–728.)* Since the lesion is restricted to the medial aspect of the basilar part of the pons, the corticospinal tract would be affected, producing paralysis of the contralateral limbs. Although other structures would also be affected and could produce additional deficits, such deficits are not listed in this question. The other dysfunctions listed would not occur because they are associated with structures situated in the pontine tegmentum, which is not included in this lesion.

**270. The answer is c.** *(Kandel, 3/e, pp 728–729.)* The lesion involves the superior colliculus. This structure receives inputs from the cerebral cortex and optic tract and its neurons respond to moving objects in the visual field. It is considered essential for the regulation of tracking movements. Lesions of the superior colliculus have not been shown to produce any of the other deficits listed in this question. Nystagmus is not likely to occur because the lesion does not involve the medial longitudinal fasciculus or the pontine gaze center.

**271. The answer is a.** *(Kandel, 3/e, pp 728–729.)* The lesion will disrupt fibers of the medial lemniscus (lateral aspect of the lesion) and thus produce contralateral loss of conscious proprioception. It will also disrupt fibers passing from the cerebellum to the red nucleus and ventrolateral (VL) nucleus of the thalamus, which could account for a tremor of the contralateral limb. Note that there would be no ipsilateral motor loss because functions associated with the red nucleus are expressed on the contralateral side. Oculomotor palsy would also be present because the lesion disrupts root fibers of cranial nerve III. However, the lesion is too rostral to affect cranial nerve IV. There is no hearing loss because the auditory fibers are situated too far laterally. Since the taste pathway is essentially ipsilateral, if any fibers are damaged by the lesion, deficits in taste sensation would be ipsilateral.

**272. The answer is c.** *(Kandel, 3/e, p 728.)* The primary structures damaged by this lesion include the crus cerebri, which results in an upper motor neuron paralysis of the contralateral limbs as well as a paresis of the lower facial and tongue muscles. The other outstanding syndrome present from this lesion is a paralysis that results from damage to cranial nerve III. Other structures may be marginally affected.

**273. The answer is a.** *(Cooper, 7/e, pp 293–297.)* The pars compacta of the substantia nigra contains dopamine neurons whose axons project to the neostriatum. In contrast, the dopaminergic neurons of the ventral tegmental area project to other areas of the forebrain, such as the hypothalamus, limbic system, and cerebral cortex. There is no known overlap in the distribution of these dopaminergic projection systems. A Parkinsonian-like syndrome results from damage to the pars compacta of the substantia nigra, but not from a lesion restricted to the ventral tegmental region.

**274. The answer is b.** *(Nolte, 3/e, pp 215–218.)* The principal ascending pathway of the auditory system listed in this question is the lateral lemniscus. It transmits information from the cochlear nuclei to the inferior colliculus. The trapezoid body is a commissure that contains some of the fibers of the lateral lemniscus that cross from the cochlear nuclei of one side of the brainstem en route to the inferior colliculus of the other side. The trapezoid body is present at the level of the caudal pons. The brachium of the superior colliculus, trigeminal lemniscus, and medial lemniscus do not transmit auditory sensory information.

# SENSORY SYSTEMS

## Questions

**DIRECTIONS:** Each group of questions below consists of lettered headings followed by a set of numbered items. For each numbered item select the **one** lettered heading with which it is **most** closely associated. Each lettered heading may be used **once, more than once, or not at all.**

### Questions 275–277

Match each description with the appropriate structure.

a. Bipolar cells
b. Ganglion cells
c. Rods
d. Cones
e. Optic nerve fibers
f. Horizontal cells

**275.** Processes arising from ganglion cells

**276.** A direct interneuron between receptor and ganglion cell

**277.** Structure associated with daylight vision

### Questions 278–280

Match each description with the appropriate structure.

a. Horizontal cells
b. Bipolar cells
c. Ganglion cells
d. Amacrine cells
e. Cones
f. Rods

**278.** Detectors of dim light

**279.** Structures that produce action potentials

**280.** Processes that are capable of depolarizing photoreceptor cells

## Questions 281–283

Match each lens below with the visual defect it corrects.

a. Emmetropia
b. Hyperopia
c. Glaucoma
d. Presbyopia
e. Astigmatism
f. Cataract
g. Myopia

**281.** Cylindrical lens

**282.** Concave spherical lens

**283.** Convex lens

## Questions 284–287

Match each irregularity with the visual defect it causes.

a. Hyperopia
b. Cataract
c. Glaucoma
d. Presbyopia
e. Astigmatism
f. Myopia

**284.** Oblong shape of the cornea or lens

**285.** Increased intraocular pressure

**286.** Denaturation and coagulation of proteins of lens

**287.** Focus of light in front of the retina

## Questions 288–290

Match each lesion with the correct visual defect.

a. Left homonymous hemianopsia
b. Right homonymous hemianopsia
c. Bitemporal hemianopsia
d. Blindness in the right eye
e. Blindness in the left eye
f. Lower right quadrantanopia

**288.** Lesion of the right optic nerve

**289.** Lesion of the right optic tract

**290.** Lesion of the optic chiasm

## Questions 291–293

Match each lesion with the appropriate visual defect.

a. Upper left quadrantanopia
b. Lower left quadrantanopia
c. Upper right quadrantanopia
d. Lower right quadrantanopia
e. Blindness in the right eye
f. Bitemporal hemianopsia

**291.** Lesion of the right temporal lobe

**292.** Lesion of the right superior bank of the calcarine fissure

**293.** Lesion of the right inferior bank of the calcarine fissure

**DIRECTIONS:**    Each question below contains five suggested responses. Select the **one best** response to each question.

**294.** The conscious perception of movement is mediated by which of the following receptors?

a. Meissner's corpuscles
b. Free nerve endings
c. Merkel's receptors
d. Joint capsules
e. Pacinian corpuscles

**295.** Which of the following types of inhibition have been identified within the dorsal column nuclei?

a. Feed forward inhibition utilizing local interneurons only
b. Feedback inhibition utilizing local interneurons only
c. Distal inhibition from fibers arising in the cerebral cortex only
d. Feed forward, feedback, and distal inhibition
e. Feed forward and distal inhibition only

**296.** Neurons capable of responding to the direction or orientation of a given stimulus moved along a receptive field are located in the

a. Spinal cord
b. Medulla
c. Pons
d. Thalamus
e. Cerebral cortex

**297.** Differentiate rapidly adapting and slowly adapting receptors.

a. A rapidly adapting receptor responds continuously to the presence of a stimulus, while a slowly adapting receptor responds only at the onset of the stimulus
b. A rapidly adapting receptor responds only at the onset of the stimulus and to any step change in the stimulus position, while the slowly adapting receptor displays a persistent response to the presence of the stimulus
c. A rapidly adapting receptor will not respond to any subsequent stimulus following the initial stimulus, while the slowly adapting receptor responds quite readily to a second stimulus
d. A rapidly adapting receptor will discharge at a high frequency to the initial stimulus and then continue to discharge but at a somewhat lower rate, while a slowly adapting receptor will discharge at a high frequency throughout the period of the duration of the stimulus
e. Rapidly adapting receptors are limited to muscle spindles, while slowly adapting receptors include those associated with pain and temperature pathways

**298.** Referred pain is the result of

a. Inhibitory fibers that block transmission of pain impulses along a given pathway and then transfer the impulses to a different pathway associated with a different part of the body
b. A massive discharge along a given pathway that results in the activation of a separate pathway because of the principle of divergence
c. A convergence of primary afferent fibers from a given region onto second-order neurons that normally receive primary afferents from a different body part
d. The disruption of lateral spinothalamic fibers
e. The blockade of substance P from primary afferent terminals

**299.** The terminals of different classes of primary nociceptive afferents have been shown to release which of the following transmitters onto dorsal horn neurons of the spinal cord?

a. Enkephalins alone
b. Glutamate alone
c. Substance P alone
d. Glutamate and substance P
e. Enkephalins, substance P, and glutamate

**300.** Stimulation of gray matter around the cerebral aqueduct and fourth ventricle can produce analgesia. This phenomenon is explained in terms of

a. Activation of a pathway that ascends directly to the cortex and mediates analgesia
b. A descending pathway that blocks nociceptive inputs at the level of the dorsal horn
c. Activation of local interneurons that block ascending nociceptive signals at the level of the midbrain
d. Activation of an ascending inhibitory pathway that projects to the ventral posterolateral (VPL) nucleus of the thalamus
e. Activation of cholinergic neurons in the basal forebrain

**301.** A cell that responds with an "on-center" and "off-surround" to generate contrast within the receptive field can be identified in

a. Retina (ganglion cell)
b. Lateral geniculate nucleus
c. Retina (ganglion cell) and lateral geniculate nucleus
d. Layer 4 of the primary visual cortex (area 17)
e. Retina (ganglion cell), lateral geniculate nucleus, and area 18

**302.** The descending pathway for central control of nociception includes

a. Fibers from the periaqueductal gray that synapse directly on dorsal horn cells
b. Fibers from the periaqueductal gray that synapse on neurons of the nucleus raphe magnus that then synapse on dorsal horn cells
c. Fibers from the periaqueductal gray that synapse upon inferior olivary neurons that then synapse upon dorsal horn cells
d. Hypothalamic fibers that synapse upon neurons of the nucleus solitarius that then synapse upon neurons of the dorsal horn
e. Hypothalamic fibers that synapse directly upon dorsal horn neurons

**303.** Fibers in each optic tract synapse in

a. The lateral geniculate nucleus only
b. The lateral geniculate nucleus and the pretectal area
c. The lateral geniculate nucleus, the pretectal area, and the superior colliculus
d. The lateral geniculate nucleus, the pretectal area, the superior colliculus, and the suprachiasmatic nucleus
e. The lateral geniculate nucleus, the pretectal area, the superior colliculus, the suprachiasmatic nucleus, and the nuclei of cranial nerves III and IV

**304.** At the level of the dorsal horn of the spinal cord, nociceptive transmission may be blocked when descending fibers are

a. Opioidergic and only contact dendrites of postsynaptic neurons that contain opiate receptors
b. Opioidergic and only contact opiate receptors located presynaptically on nociceptive terminals
c. Opioidergic and contact both dendrites of postsynaptic neurons and presynaptic terminals, both of which contain opiate receptors
d. Serotonergic and only contact dendrites of postsynaptic neurons that contain 5-HT receptors
e. Cholinergic and contact both dendrites of postsynaptic neurons and presynaptic terminals, both of which contain muscarinic receptors

**305.** In the olfactory glomerulus, primary afferent fibers terminate principally upon

a. Granule cell dendrites forming axodendritic synapses
b. Granule cell axon terminals forming axoaxonic synapses
c. Mitral cell dendrites forming axodendritic synapses
d. Mitral cell axon terminals forming axoaxonic synapses
e. Axon terminals of fibers arising from the olfactory tubercle, forming axoaxonic synapses

**306.** When a cone is hyperpolarized by light,

a. The "on-center" bipolar cell is excited and the "off-center" bipolar cell is inhibited
b. The "on-center" bipolar cell will inhibit the ganglion cell with which it makes synaptic contact
c. The ganglion cell that receives its input from an "off-center" bipolar cell will discharge because the bipolar cell is excited during the presence of the stimulus
d. An "on-center" bipolar cell excites a neighboring ganglion cell that receives its input from an "off-center" bipolar cell
e. Transmitter released from a cone cell has the same effect upon all processes with which it synapses

**307.** The region of the cortex most closely associated with the conscious perception of smell is the

a. Temporal neocortex
b. Posterior parietal lobule
c. Cingulate gyrus
d. Prefrontal cortex
e. Precentral gyrus

**308.** Lateral inhibition within the retina is most effectively achieved through the action of

a. Rod cells
b. Cone cells
c. Bipolar cells
d. Ganglion cells
e. Horizontal cells

**309.** Cells that respond to an image in a specific position and have discrete excitatory and inhibitory zones and a specific axis of orientation in which a response occurs are classified as

a. M cells of the lateral geniculate nucleus
b. P cells of the lateral geniculate nucleus
c. Simple cells of the visual cortex
d. Complex cells of the visual cortex
e. Hypercomplex cells of the visual cortex

**310.** The part of the olfactory receptor mechanism that initially responds to an olfactory stimulus is the

a. Mitral cell
b. Granule cell
c. Sustentacular cell
d. Basal cell
e. Olfactory cilia

**311.** The neural basis of olfactory discrimination is believed to utilize

a. Specific activation of different cell groups within the amygdala
b. Specific activation of different groups of olfactory glomeruli that are spatially organized and segregated within the olfactory bulb
c. Specific activation of different groups of cells within the olfactory tubercle
d. Temporal summation of olfactory signals in the anterior olfactory nucleus
e. Temporal summation of olfactory signals in the mediodorsal thalamic nucleus

**312.** The principal efferent pathway of the olfactory bulb arises from

a. Granule cells
b. Golgi cells
c. Receptor cells
d. Mitral cells
e. Periglomerular cells

**313.** Direct efferent projections of the olfactory bulb supply the

a. Hypothalamus and prefrontal cortex
b. Amygdala and pyriform cortex
c. Hippocampus and amygdala
d. Prefrontal cortex and medial thalamus
e. Septal area and prefrontal cortex

**314.** Which of the following statements concerning "uncinate fits" is correct?

a. They are characterized by olfactory hallucinations that occur as a result of an irritating lesion of the uncus, adjoining region of the parahippocampal gyrus, or region adjoining the amygdala
b. They are characterized by olfactory hallucinations that occur as a result of an irritating lesion of the mediodorsal thalamic nucleus
c. They are an epileptic disorder whose focus is the prefrontal cortex, and they result in a failure to discriminate odors
d. They are a partial complex seizure disorder of the amygdala and hippocampus that results in the expression of violent, uncontrolled behavior
e. They are an epileptogenic disturbance caused by the formation of a tumor that is limited to the olfactory bulb, and they result in a failure to discriminate odors

**315.** Which of the following statements about the taste system is correct?

a. Receptors for specific taste stimuli are positioned on specific regions of the tongue
b. A given taste bud will only respond to a single taste modality
c. All taste afferent fibers are contained within the facial nerve
d. The cellular mechanism for transduction is essentially the same for each of the categories of taste stimuli
e. Single primary taste fibers in the chorda tympani respond to more than one taste stimulus

**316.** Which of the following sensory systems is able to utilize a circuit that bypasses the thalamus for the transmission of sensory information from the periphery to the cerebral cortex?

a. Conscious proprioception
b. Taste
c. Olfaction
d. Vision
e. Audition

# SENSORY SYSTEMS

## Answers

**275–277. The answers are: 275-e, 276-a, 277-d.** (*Guyton, 2/e, pp 164–165. Kandel, 3/e, pp 400–410.*) The ganglion cells give rise to optic nerve fibers (E) that project to central nervous system structures that include the lateral geniculate body, pretectal region, and superior colliculus. Bipolar cells (A) serve as interneurons between the photoreceptor cell and the ganglion cell. Cones (D) are concentrated in the region of the fovea and are associated with day vision. On the other hand, rods are located elsewhere on the retina and are associated with night vision.

**278–280. The answers are: 278-f, 279-c, 280-a.** (*Guyton, 2/e, pp 164–165. Kandel, 3/e, pp 400–410, 412–415.*) Rod cells (F) are located throughout the retina and are associated with night vision because their receptive mechanisms are more sensitive to light than are cones. Cones are located in the foveal region and are associated with day vision. Within the retina, ganglion cells (C) are unique in that they are capable of initiating action potentials. Other cells in the retina do not have this capability. Horizontal cells (A) are of importance because they synapse with receptor cells. For this reason, they are capable of depolarizing receptor cells.

**281–283. The answers are: 281-e, 282-g, 283-b**. (*Guyton, 2/e, pp 144–151.*) Myopia (G) can be corrected with a concave lens. In astigmatism (E), the shape of the cornea (and possibly the lens) becomes oblong, resulting in differences in the curvature of the lens along the long and short axes. Astigmatism is corrected with a cylindrical lens. In hyperopia (B), a person has a weak lens system and light rays focus behind the retina. It is corrected with a convex lens.

**284–287. The answers are: 284-e, 285-c, 286-b, 287-f.** (*Guyton, 2/e, pp 144–151.*) Astigmatism (E) is a defect that results from the oblong shape of the cornea or lens. It is corrected with a convex lens. Glaucoma (C) is a condition of elevated intraocular pressure caused (perhaps by infection) when debris accumulates in the spaces that lead to the canal of Schlemm. If not treated, it can rapidly lead to blindness because the pressure can block conduction along the optic nerve. Cataracts (B) will occur as a result of the denaturing of proteins in the lens fibers. These proteins eventually coagulate, resulting in an opaque lens. When light rays are focused in front of the retina, myopia (F) results. This is usually due to the fact that the eyeball is too long, but may also result when the lens system of the eye has too much power.

**288–290. The answers are: 288-d, 289-a, 290-c.** *(Kandel, 3/e, pp 436–438. Nolte, 3/e, p 303.)* A lesion of the right optic nerve will produce total blindness of the right eye (D) because it damages all the retinal ganglion cell axons from that eye before any of them can cross at the optic chiasm. A lesion of the right optic tract will damage all the fibers that are associated with the left visual fields from both eyes. Accordingly, such a lesion will produce a left homonymous hemianopsia (A). A lesion of the optic chiasm will destroy the fibers that cross in the chiasm and are associated with the nasal retinal fields. Hence, such a lesion will cause a bitemporal hemianopsia (C).

**291–293. The answers are: 291-a, 292-b, 293-a.** *(Kandel, 3/e, pp 436–438. Nolte, 3/e, p 303.)* A lesion of the right temporal lobe will damage the fibers contained in the loop of Meyer. These are fibers that pass from the lateral geniculate body to the inferior bank of the calcarine fissure on the right side. However, these fibers follow a more ventral trajectory that involves parts of the temporal lobe. Since the left visual fields are located on the right side of the brain, damage to these fibers will result in an upper left quadrantanopia (A). Because the lower visual fields are represented on the superior bank of the calcarine fissure, a lesion of this region will result in a lower left quadrantanopia (B).

**294. The answer is d.** *(Nolte, 3/e, pp 101–112.)* Meissner's corpuscles, Merkel's receptors, and pacinian corpuscles respond to tactile, pressure, or possibly vibratory stimuli, while free nerve endings are associated with nociceptive stimuli. Joint capsules respond to movement of the limb, and the axons of these receptors contribute to the dorsal column–medial lemniscal system mediating the conscious perception of movement.

**295. The answer is d.** *(Kandel, 3/e, pp 368–370.)* To generate an excitatory focus with an inhibitory surround, three types of inhibition are present in the dorsal column nuclei. First-order neurons ascending in the dorsal columns make synaptic contact with different cells in the dorsal column nuclei and excite those cells. One such cell may be an inhibitory interneuron that makes synaptic contact with a neighboring dorsal column nuclear cell, thus inhibiting that cell (i.e., feed forward inhibition). In addition, the dorsal column cell that is excited by the first-order neuron may make synaptic contact with another inhibitory interneuron (in addition to its classical ascending projection to the ventral posterolateral nucleus [VPL] of the thalamus). This inhibitory interneuron makes synaptic contact with an adjacent dorsal column cell and inhibits that cell (i.e., feedback inhibition). Finally, a descending fiber from the postcentral gyrus can make synaptic contact with inhibitory interneurons that inhibit dorsal column cells. The figure below illustrates feedback, feed forward, and descending inhibition. Inhibitory neurons are depicted in black.

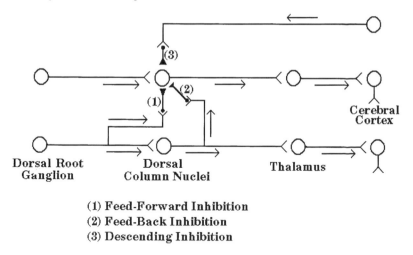

(1) **Feed-Forward Inhibition**
(2) **Feed-Back Inhibition**
(3) **Descending Inhibition**

**296. The answer is e.** *(Kandel, 3/e, pp 378–381.)* As a general rule, neurons situated in the cortex in association with any of the sensory systems take on a much higher level of complexity than neurons situated at lower levels of the relay network. In the case of the somatosensory system, direction-sensitive cells in the somatosensory cortex will respond to one direction of movement of a stimulus along the receptive field and not to another direction. Orientation-sensitive neurons respond best to movement along one axis of the receptive field. This is not true of neurons situated in lower levels of the somatosensory pathway.

**297. The answer is b.** *(Kandel, 3/e, pp 336–338.)* A rapidly adapting receptor is one that discharges initially to the presence of a stimulus and to any stepwise change in the position or intensity of that stimulus (such as when the stimulus is terminated). A slowly adapting receptor responds continuously (perhaps with a decrease in its frequency) to the presence of the stimulus. A pacinian corpuscle is an example of a rapidly adapting receptor; axons from this receptor contribute to the dorsal column–medial lemniscal system.

**298. The answer is c.** *(Kandel, 3/e, pp 388–389.)* Referred pain is a phenomenon in which pain impulses, arising from primary afferent fibers from one part of the body (such as from deep visceral structures), terminate on dorsal horn projection neurons that normally receive cutaneous afferents from a different part of the body (such as the arm). In this situation, a person who is suffering a heart attack experiences pain that appears to be coming from the arm. It is the convergence of these distinctly different inputs onto the same projection neurons that provides the basis for this phenomenon. None of the other possible mechanisms listed in this question have an anatomic or physiologic basis.

**299. The answer is d.** *(Kandel, 3/e, pp 389–390.)* Primary nociceptive afferent fibers would have to release an excitatory transmitter in order for normal transmission to take place. Two excitatory transmitters have been identified in association with different classes of primary nociceptive afferents: substance P and excitatory amino acids. The best candidate as an excitatory amino acid is glutamate. Since enkephalins have been shown to be inhibitory transmitters in the pain system, they are not likely to be released from the primary afferents. Instead, other central nervous system neurons impinge upon the primary afferents and enkephalins are released from those neurons.

**300. The answer is b.** *(Kandel, 3/e, pp 392–394.)* Perhaps one of the most important discoveries in pain research made over the past 15 years is of a descending pathway that originates in the midbrain periaqueductal gray and makes synaptic contacts in the medulla. From the medulla this pathway descends to the dorsal horn, where these fibers provide the anatomic substrate for suppression of pain inputs that enter the spinal cord from the periphery. There are no known inputs to the cortex that directly produce analgesia. The mechanism governing analgesia appears to operate at lower brainstem and spinal cord levels. The ascending fibers for transmission of pain impulses reach thalamic nuclei directly and, thus, local interneurons within the midbrain would not be able to interfere with such transmission. The pathway to the ventral posterolateral (VPL) nucleus of the thalamus is an excitatory one and is not known to have any inhibitory properties. Cholinergic neurons in the basal forebrain have been implicated in memory functions and are not known to have any role in the regulation of pain sensation.

**301. The answer is c.** (*Kandel, 3/e, pp 410–430.*) Both retina ganglion cells and lateral geniculate neurons exhibit an "on-center" and "off-surround" with respect to objects in the receptive field. Cells in area 18 of the visual cortex are not known to possess these characteristics. Cells in layer 4 of the primary visual cortex do not have circular receptive fields. Instead, these cells respond to such stimuli as lines and bars.

**302. The answer is b.** (*Kandel, 3/e, pp 393–394.*) The descending pathway for central inhibition of nociception involves the following: Fibers that originate in the midbrain periaqueductal gray matter project caudally to the level of the nucleus raphe magnus, upon whose neurons they synapse. Fibers from the nucleus raphe magnus then project further caudally, where they synapse in the dorsal horn of the spinal cord.

**303. The answer is d.** (*Guyton, 2/e, pp 157–168.*) Fibers of the optic tract synapse in a number of regions associated with the processing of visual information or visual reflex activity. These include the lateral geniculate nuclei (part of the classical visual pathway for relaying visual information to the visual cortex), the pretectal area (for elicitation of the pupillary light reflex and reflex movements of the eyes), the superior colliculus (for bilateral control of rapid eye movements), and the suprachiasmatic nucleus (which relates to the control of circadian rhythms). There are no known monosynaptic projections from the retina to the nuclei of cranial nerves III and IV.

**304. The answer is c.** (*Kandel, 3/e, pp 396–397.*) Evidence indicates that within the dorsal horn of the spinal cord, descending pain inhibitory fibers from the lower brainstem (serotonergic and noradrenergic fibers) synapse upon interneurons that are enkephalinergic. These enkephalinergic neurons then synapse upon both presynaptic terminals of primary pain afferent fibers and the dendrites of dorsal horn projection neurons (which also receive inputs from the primary nociceptive afferent fibers).

**305. The answer is c.** (*Guyton, 2/e, pp 191–193. Kandel, 3/e, pp 515–517. Nolte, 3/e, pp 393–395.*) The olfactory receptor and its primary afferent fiber terminate upon dendrites of mitral cells. This relationship is of importance because it is the axon of the mitral cell that projects out of the olfactory bulb (forming the major component of the lateral olfactory stria). The granule cell processes make synaptic contact with dendrites of mitral cells, forming dendrodendritic synapses, but are not known to make synaptic contact with primary afferent terminals. Cells arising in the olfactory tubercle are not known to project to the olfactory bulb. Instead, projections of cells situated in the olfactory tubercle contribute fibers to the medial forebrain bundle and stria medullaris.

**306. The answer is a.** (*Kandel, 3/e, pp 413–415.*) When a cone is hyperpolarized by light there is a reduction in the release of transmitter substance (glutamate). This reduced amount of transmitter results in excitation of the "on-center" bipolar cell and inhibition of the "off-center" bipolar cell (presumably because the two types of bipolar cells contain different postsynaptic receptors). Since bipolar cells excite the ganglion cells, an "off-center" bipolar cell will be inhibited when light is present and, thus, will be unable to excite the ganglion cell to which it is connected. "On-center" bipolar cells are excited when light is present and so are the ganglion cells to which they are connected. In addition, "on-center" bipolar cells inhibit ganglion cells that receive their primary input from "off-center" bipolar cells. This serves to increase the likelihood that these ganglion cells will remain inhibited when the light stimulus is present. A cone cell may make synaptic contact with two types of bipolar cells ("on-center" or "off-center"). Because they possess different postsynaptic receptor mechanisms, the two types of bipolar cells will respond differently to input from cones.

**307. The answer is d.** *(Kandel, 3/e, pp 517–518.)* Experimental evidence indicates the prefrontal cortex is a key region for the conscious perception of smell. This conclusion is based upon two observations. First, the prefrontal cortex receives major inputs from the olfactory bulb by following routes: olfactory bulb to pyriform cortex to prefrontal cortex; or olfactory bulb to pyriform cortex (and olfactory tubercle) to mediodorsal thalamic nucleus to prefrontal cortex. Second, lesions of the prefrontal cortex result in a failure to discriminate odors. Olfactory functions are not known to be associated with any of the other choices. Instead, the primary auditory receiving area is located in the auditory cortex; the posterior parietal lobule is concerned with such processes as the programming mechanisms associated with complex motor tasks; the cingulate gyrus has been associated with such functions as spatial learning and the modulation of autonomic and emotional processes; and the prefrontal gyrus contains the primary motor area.

**308. The answer is e.** *(Kandel, 3/e, pp 409–415.)* Lateral inhibition within the retina is generated most effectively by the horizontal cells. A horizontal cell receives inputs from a given receptor cell and, when activated, inhibits adjacent receptor cells. It is possible for a given cone cell to differentially affect two neighboring bipolar cells and for an "oncenter" bipolar cell to hyperpolarize an adjacent "offcenter" ganglion cell. However, the primary flow of information through these neuronal elements is in the plane of orientation that most directly connects the receptor cell to the ganglion cell through a bipolar cell. Therefore, the contribution of these elements to lateral inhibition is relatively minimal (if at all) in comparison to the effects generated by horizontal cells. The ganglion cell is not known to play any role in lateral inhibition.

**309. The answer is c.** *(Guyton, 2/e, pp 169–171. Kandel, 3/e, pp 426–431.)* Cells in the lateral geniculate nucleus respond very much like ganglion cells in the retina because of the point-to-point projection pathway from the retina to the lateral geniculate. Accordingly, lateral geniculate cells have small concentric receptive fields that are either oncenter or offcenter in which the cells respond best to small spots of light that are in the center of the receptive field. On the other hand, cells in the visual cortex display a much greater complexity in their responses to images in the visual field. Instead of responding to small spots of light, they respond to lines and borders in the different areas of the visual field. In particular, the simple cell responds as a function of the retinal position in which the line stimulus is located as well as its orientation (e.g., whether it is in a vertical or horizontal position). As a result, when a bar of light is positioned in the appropriate part of the visual field with the appropriate orientation, the cells in area 17 will respond maximally. When either of these parameters is altered, the firing pattern of the cell will be reduced or totally inhibited. Complex cells lack clear excitatory and inhibitory zones (i.e., these neurons respond to bars of light in a given orientation but they are not position-specific). Hypercomplex cells are stimulated by bars of light of specific lengths or by specific shapes.

**310. The answer is e.** *(Guyton, 2/e, pp 191–192. Kandel, 3/e, pp 312–314.)* The olfactory cilia are extensions of the receptor cell and it is this part of the cell that initially responds to an olfactory stimulus. The cilia contain protein membranes that bind with different odorants, which constitutes a necessary condition for excitation of the olfactory cell. Mitral and granule cells are situated in the olfactory bulb and, consequently, are not part of the receptor mechanism. Sustentacular cells are supporting cells and are not part of the receptor mechanism. Basal cells are the precursor cells for receptor cells and, thus, are also not directly part of the receptor mechanism.

**311. The answer is b.** *(Guyton, 2/e, p 193. Kandel, 3/e, pp 516–518.)* A number of recent studies have indicated that different olfactory glomeruli respond to different kinds of olfactory stimuli. In a sense this represents a type of organization of the olfactory bulb that bears a functional similarity to the spatial organization that exists for other sensory systems. There is no evidence that such a spatial arrangement exists for other components of the olfactory system, nor is there any evidence that temporal summation plays any role in the process of olfactory discrimination.

**312. The answer is d.** *(Nolte, 3/e, pp 394–397.)* The principal output pathways of the olfactory bulb arise from mitral cells and a related cell called tufted cells. The mitral cells project their axons out of the olfactory bulb to other regions of the forebrain associated with the transmission of olfactory information to the cerebral cortex. The major pathway subserving this is the lateral olfactory stria. Other cells that are mentioned in this question are either not present in the olfactory bulb (Golgi cells) or they have no known projections outside of the olfactory bulb. Receptor cells project only as far as the glomerulus. The granule cell has no axon. The periglomerular cell makes only local connections among neighboring glomeruli.

**313. The answer is b.** *(Kandel, 3/e, p 518. Nolte, 3/e, pp 393–394.)* Mitral cell axons enter the lateral olfactory stria and project caudally through this bundle to supply the medial amygdala and pyriform cortex. Olfactory projections to other nuclei such as the hippocampal formation, prefrontal cortex, medial thalamus, and septal area require at least one additional synaptic connection such as in the pyriform cortex, amygdala, or olfactory tubercle.

**314. The answer is a.** *(Kandel, 3/e, p 518. Nolte, 3/e, pp 397.)* Uncinate fits are characterized by seizure activity involving portions of the anterior aspect of the temporal lobe. The structures most often implicated include the uncus, parahippocampal gyrus, the region of the amygdala and adjoining tissue, and the pyriform cortex. During the occurrence of uncinate fits, a person experiences olfactory hallucinations of a highly unpleasant nature.

**315. The answer is e.** *(Kandel, 3/e, pp 521–525.)* A primary afferent fiber innervates many taste receptors. Recordings from the primary afferent fiber reveal that it responds to different modalities of taste stimuli, although it may preferentially respond to a single, given modality. This would suggest that taste discrimination and perception occur as a result of the comparison of the activation pattern of different groups of taste fibers. Different types of taste receptors may be positioned in the same region of the tongue. Primary afferent taste fibers respond to more than one modality of taste stimuli. Taste fibers from the anterior two thirds of the tongue are carried in the facial nerve; fibers from the posterior third of the tongue are carried in the glossopharyngeal nerve, and taste fibers from the epiglottis are carried in the vagus nerve. The cellular mechanism for transduction of taste stimuli depends upon the stimulus. For example, receptors for molecules associated with sweet and bitter tastes utilize second messengers, while those associated with sour and salty tasting molecules act directly upon the ion channels.

**316. The answer is c.** *(Nolte, 3/e, pp 134–138, 187–193, 393–397, 399–410.)* The pathway for conscious proprioception from the body utilizes the ventral posterolateral nucleus as its thalamic relay. Conscious proprioception from the head utilizes the ventral posteromedial (VPM) nucleus as its relay. The taste pathway utilizes the VPM nucleus as well. The visual system utilizes the lateral geniculate nucleus, and the auditory system utilizes the medial geniculate nucleus. In contrast, the olfactory system can transmit olfactory information to the prefrontal cortex without engaging thalamic nuclei. Thus, olfactory information reaches the pyriform cortex and amygdala from the olfactory bulb and then is transmitted directly to the prefrontal cortex. However, it should be noted that olfactory information also can reach the prefrontal cortex by virtue of projections from the olfactory tubercle and pyriform cortex via the mediodorsal thalamic nucleus. Thus, the olfactory system may utilize a parallel processing mechanism in transmitting inputs to the prefrontal cortex.

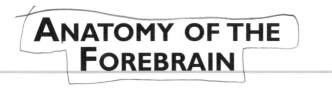

# ANATOMY OF THE FOREBRAIN

## Questions

**DIRECTIONS:** Each group of questions below consists of lettered points on a diagram followed by a set of numbered items. For each numbered item select the **one** point on the diagram with which it is **most** closely associated. Each lettered point may be used **once, more than once, or not at all.**

**Questions 317–321**

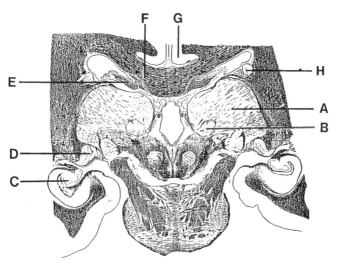

(Adapted from Villiger, Fig. 27; with permission.)

**317.** Neurons in this region project their axons to the inferior parietal lobule

**318.** This fiber bundle arises from the hippocampal formation

**319.** A lesion of this structure produces short-term memory deficits

**320.** This is a specific relay nucleus

**321.** Neurons in this region innervate the striatum

## Questions 322–329

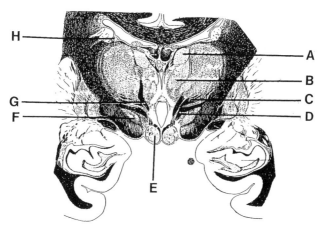

(Adapted from Villiger, Fig. 34; with permission.)

**322.** This structure has pallidal fibers that project to the ventrolateral (VL) and ventral anterior (VA) nuclei of the thalamus

**323.** This nucleus maintains reciprocal connections with the globus pallidus

**324.** This structure receives fibers from the mamillary bodies

**325.** These fibers project to the medial hypothalamus

**326.** This structure contains fibers that arise from both the pallidum and cerebellum

**327.** This region receives inputs from the hippocampal formation and projects its axons to the anterior thalamic nucleus

**328.** These fibers arise from the mamillary bodies

**329.** This region has reciprocal connections with large parts of the frontal lobe

## Questions 330–336

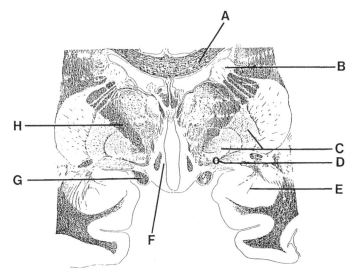

(Adapted from Villiger, Fig. 38; with permission.)

**330.** These fibers arise from layers V-VI of cerebral cortex

**331.** These fibers arise from layers II-III of cerebral cortex

**332.** These fibers arise from the globus pallidus

**333.** This region receives dopaminergic inputs from the substantia nigra

**334.** Cells in this region produce hormones that are released in the posterior pituitary

**335.** This structure powerfully modulates hypothalamic functions

**336.** A lesion of this structure will produce a hemianopsia

**Questions 337–341**

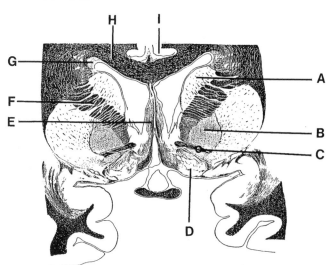

(Adapted from Villiger, Fig. 44; with permission.)

**337.** This structure receives afferent fibers from the cerebral cortex and thalamus

**338.** This structure is the source of a major cholinergic projection to the neocortex

**339.** This structure receives inputs from the neostriatum

**340.** This structure transmits olfactory information from the anterior olfactory nucleus

**341.** This structure (which is considerably larger in nonhumans such as rat, cat, and monkey) is a component of the limbic system and receives a major afferent projection from the hippocampal formation

# ANATOMY OF THE FOREBRAIN

## *Answers*

**317–321. The answers are: 317-a, 318-e, 319-c, 320-d, 321-b.**
*(Noback, 5/e, p 336. Nolte, 3/e, pp 250–251, 285–289, 400–408.)* This section
is taken at the level of the posterior thalamus and, because of the oblique
cut, also includes parts of the midbrain and pons. The fornix (E), situated
just below the corpus callosum, arises from the hippocampal formation and
supplies the septal area, anterior thalamic nucleus, and the mamillary bodies. The hippocampal formation (C) is associated with a number of different processes including short-term memory. Thus, a lesion of this structure
will likely produce deficits in short-term memory. The lateral geniculate nucleus (D), situated in the far ventrolateral aspect of the posterior thalamus,
is a relay nucleus for the transmission of visual information to the cortex.
The centromedian nucleus (B), identified by its encapsulated appearance,
can be found in posterior levels of the thalamus, where it projects to the
neostriatum. Also located at the level of the posterior aspect of the thalamus
is the pulvinar nucleus (A). This large structure projects its axons to the inferior parietal lobule.

**322–329. The answers are; 322-d, 323-f, 324-a, 325-h, 326-c, 327-e,
328-g, 329-b.** *(Nolte, 3/e, pp 251, 258, 267–268, 323–329, 406–408.)* This
section is taken at the level of the mamillary bodies (at ventral levels) and
includes parts of the anterior thalamus (at dorsal levels). The lenticular fasciculus (D), situated just below the thalamic fasciculus and immediately
above the subthalamic nucleus at the level of this brain section, arises from
the dorsomedial aspect of the medial pallidal segment and projects to the
ventrolateral (VL), ventral anterior (VA), and centromedian (CM) nuclei of
the thalamus. Note that the thalamic fasciculus (C) also projects to these nuclei. While many of the fibers contained in this bundle arise from the pallidum, others arise directly from the cerebellum. The subthalamic nucleus
(F), which lies on the dorsal surface of the internal capsule, maintains reciprocal connections with the globus pallidus through a pathway called the

subthalamic fasciculus. The anterior nucleus of the thalamus (A), which lies at the rostral end of the thalamus in a dorsomedial position, receives a major input from the mamillary bodies via the mamillothalamic tract. The region immediately below the tail and body of the caudate nucleus is occupied by a major output pathway of the medial amygdala, the stria terminalis (H). It supplies the medial preoptic region, bed nucleus of the stria terminalis, and medial hypothalamus.

The thalamic fasciculus (C) can be seen in sections taken through the caudal half of the thalamus and is clearly visualized in a position dorsal to the subthalamic nucleus and lenticular fasciculus. It contains fibers that arise from both the dentate nucleus of the cerebellum and the medial pallidal segment. The mamillary bodies (E), situated at the base of the posterior aspect of the hypothalamus, are the origin of the mamillothalamic (G) tract, which innervates the anterior thalamic nucleus. A large nuclear mass situated in the medial aspect of the posterior two thirds of the thalamus is the mediodorsal thalamic nucleus (B). This nucleus projects extensively to wide regions of the frontal lobe, including the prefrontal cortex. In turn, the prefrontal region of cortex and adjoining regions of the frontal lobe project their axons back to the mediodorsal nucleus. Thus, there are reciprocal connections linking the mediodorsal nucleus and rostral portions of the frontal lobe.

**330–336. The answers are: 330-h, 331-a, 332-d, 333-b, 334-f, 335-e, 336-g.** (*Nolte, 3/e, pp 265–272, 323–330, 361–367.*) This section is taken from rostral levels of the diencephalon. Corticobulbar and corticospinal fibers contained within the internal capsule (H) arise from the deeper layers of cerebral cortex (i.e., layers V–VI), while those of the corpus callosum (A) arise from more superficial layers of the cortex (i.e., layers II–III) and project to the homotypic region of the contralateral cortex. Fibers of the ansa lenticularis (D) arise from the ventral aspect of the medial pallidal segment and can be visualized at more anterior levels of the pallidum. Its axons supply the ventrolateral (VL), ventral anterior (VA), and centromedian (CM) nuclei of the thalamus. The caudate nucleus (B) receives dopaminergic inputs from the substantia nigra.

Different cells of the paraventricular nucleus of the hypothalamus (F), situated in the dorsomedial region at anterior levels, synthesize oxytocin and vasopressin. These hormones are transported down their axons to the posterior pituitary. Different fiber groups of the amygdala (E) provide major inputs into the medial and lateral regions of the hypothalamus and thus constitute a significant modulator of hypothalamic functions. The optic tract (G) arises from the retina. Each optic tract represents fibers associated with the visual fields of the opposite side. Therefore, a lesion of the optic tract will result in a homonymous hemianopsia.

**337–341. The answers are: 337-a, 338-d, 339-b, 340-c, 341-e.** *(Nolte, 3/e, pp 323–331, 394, 399, 415–416.)* This section is taken at the level of the septum pellucidum, anterior commissure, and the substantia innominata. Fibers from the region of the basal nucleus of Meynert located in the substantia innominata (D) (at the base of the brain in the far rostral forebrain) send a cholinergic projection to wide areas of the neocortex. The globus pallidus (B) receives inputs from the neostriatum (i.e., caudate nucleus and putamen). The anterior commissure (C) can be clearly seen at the level of the forebrain just rostral to the level of the preoptic area. It transmits olfactory information from the anterior olfactory nucleus on one side of the brain to the olfactory bulb and anterior olfactory nucleus of the contralateral side. The septal area (E), seen at this level of the forebrain as a thin structure separated by the lateral ventricles on both sides, receives major inputs from the hippocampal formation and is a principal component of the limbic system. The caudate nucleus (A) and the putamen constitute the principal structures for receipt of afferent fibers. Primary sources of such input include the cerebral cortex and centromedian (CM) nucleus of the thalamus.

# MOTOR SYSTEMS

## Questions

**DIRECTIONS:** Each question below contains five suggested responses. Select the **one best** response to each question.

**342.** A patient delays initiation of movement, displays an uneven trajectory in moving her hand from above her head to touch her nose, and is uneven in her attempts to demonstrate rapid alternation of pronating and supernating movements of the hand and forearm. She probably has a lesion in the

a. Hemispheres of the posterior cerebellar lobe
b. Flocculonodular lobe of the cerebellum
c. Vermal region of the anterior cerebellar lobe
d. Fastigial nucleus
e. Ventral spinocerebellar tract

**343.** Spasticity may result from a lesion of

a. Ventral horn cells
b. Corpus callosum
c. Postcentral gyrus
d. Internal capsule
e. Substantia nigra

**344.** In studying the functional relationships between motor cortex and spinal cord, which of the following effects of cortical stimulation on synaptic potentials would an investigator be likely to observe?

a. The largest potentials would be seen in spinal motor neurons that innervate proximal muscles
b. The largest potentials would be seen in spinal motor neurons that innervate distal muscles
c. The potentials seen in spinal motor neurons that innervate proximal and distal muscles would be approximately equivalent
d. The largest potentials would be seen in spinal sensory neurons that carry information from spindle afferents to the cerebellum
e. The largest potentials would be seen in spinal sensory neurons that carry information from proprioceptors to the thalamus

**345.** Which of the following statements correctly characterizes properties of neurons in the motor cortex?

a. In the resting state, the membranes of motor cortex neurons are more permeable to sodium than to potassium ions
b. Motor cortex neurons receive information from the muscle to which they project or from a region of skin related to the function of that muscle
c. Motor cortex neurons have reciprocal connections with the red nucleus
d. Motor cortex neurons that excite alpha motor neurons generally have little effect upon gamma motor neurons that project to the same muscle group
e. Motor neurons of the cerebral cortex have reciprocal, monosynaptic connections with neurons in the cerebellar cortex

**346.** Paralysis of the right side of the lower face, right spastic paralysis of the limbs, deviation of the tongue to the right with no atrophy, and no loss of taste from any region of the tongue will likely result from a lesion of the

a. Internal capsule of the right side
b. Internal capsule of the left side
c. Right pontine tegmentum
d. Base of the medulla on right side
e. Base of the medulla on left side

**347.** An impairment in the ability to perform certain types of learned, complex movements (referred to as apraxia) usually results from a lesion of the

a. Precentral gyrus
b. Postcentral gyrus
c. Premotor cortex
d. Prefrontal cortex
e. Cingulate gyrus

**348.** The overwhelming majority of fibers that supply the basal ganglia terminate in the

a. Paleostriatum
b. Neostriatum
c. Subthalamic nucleus
d. Substantia nigra
e. Claustrum

**349.** Neurons in the neostriatum are

a. Inhibited by gamma-aminobutyric acid (GABA) released at corticostriate terminals
b. Inhibited by GABA released at nigrostriatal terminals
c. Inhibited by substance P released at corticostriate terminals
d. Excited by acetylcholine released from hypothalamic-caudate terminals
e. Excited by glutamate released at corticostriate terminals

**350.** The primary transmitter released from terminals of both neostriatal and paleostriatal neurons is

a.  Glycine
b.  Enkephalin
c.  Dopamine
d.  Gamma-aminobutyric acid (GABA)
e.  Glutamate

**351.** Since motor dysfunctions associated with disturbances of basal ganglia are expressed on the contralateral side of the body, one may conclude that the basal ganglia project

a.  Fibers to the spinal cord that are crossed
b.  Fibers to motor nuclei of the brainstem whose axons then project to the contralateral spinal cord
c.  Fibers to structures that ultimately influence motor regions of the ipsilateral cerebral cortex
d.  Axons to the cerebellum, whose outputs are known to modulate the contralateral side of the body
e.  Fibers directly to the contralateral motor cortex

**352.** The major afferent input to the flocculonodular lobe is from the

a.  Nucleus dorsalis of Clarke of the spinal cord
b.  Red nucleus
c.  Vestibular nuclei
d.  Cerebral cortex
e.  Midbrain reticular formation

**353.** In Huntington's disease, there is a loss of

a.  Dopamine in the neostriatum
b.  Substance P in the substantia nigra
c.  Acetylcholine and GABA in intrastriatal and cortical neurons
d.  Serotonin in the neostriatum
e.  Most of the pallidal neurons

**354.** Damage to the subthalamic nucleus will result in

a.  Torsion dystonia
b.  Tremor at rest
c.  Hemiballism
d.  Spastic paralysis
e.  Tardive dyskinesia

**355.** Which of the following drugs ameliorate choreiform movements?

a.  Acetylcholine blockers because there is an excess of this transmitter in the caudate nucleus
b.  Dopamine blockers because there is too low a ratio of acetylcholine to dopamine in the neostriatum
c.  Serotonin blockers because there is too low a ratio of serotonin to acetylcholine and dopamine in the neostriatum
d.  Substance P antagonists because the ratio of substance P to acetylcholine is too high in the neostriatum
e.  Norepinephrine antagonists because the ratio of norepinephrine to acetylcholine is too high in the subthalamic nucleus

**356.** Tardive dyskinesia is most likely the result of

a. A change in serotonin receptors that causes a hypersensitivity to serotonin
b. A change in acetylcholine receptors that causes a hypersensitivity to acetylcholine
c. A change in enkephalin receptors that causes a hypersensitivity to enkephalin
d. A change in dopamine receptors that causes a hypersensitivity to dopamine
e. A change in GABA receptors that causes hypersensitivity to GABA

**357.** The neurotoxin MPTP (1-methyl-4-phenyl-1, 2, 3, 6-tetrahydropyridine) has recently been applied experimentally with considerable success as a model for

a. Huntington's disease
b. Hemiballism
c. Parkinson's disease
d. Tardive dyskinesia
e. Dystonia

**358.** The dorsal spinocerebellar tract, the ventral spinocerebellar tract, and the cuneocerebellar tract, in a general sense, show convergence in their projections to the cerebellum. The principal region within the cerebellum where these fibers converge is the

a. Anterior lobe
b. Posterior lobe
c. Flocculonodular lobe
d. Fastigial nucleus
e. Dentate nucleus

**359.** Information arising from the cerebral cortex is known to reach the cerebellum. The fibers carrying it are

a. Somatotopically distributed only to the anterior lobe
b. Somatotopically distributed only to the vermal region of the anterior and posterior lobes
c. Somatotopically distributed to the cerebellar hemispheres
d. Not somatotopically organized but do project to the hemispheres of the anterior and posterior lobes
e. Distributed mainly to the interposed and dentate nuclei

**360.** A cerebellar glomerulus includes

a. Mossy fiber terminals, Golgi axons, and axon terminals of granule cells
b. Climbing fiber terminals, Golgi axons, and granule cell dendrites
c. Mossy fiber terminals, Purkinje cell axons, and granule cell dendrites
d. Mossy fiber terminals, Golgi and granule cell dendrites, and Golgi cell axon terminals
e. Climbing fiber terminals, Golgi cell dendrites, Purkinje cell dendrites, and axon terminals of parallel fibers

## Questions 361–363

The cerebellum contains a number of important feedback relationships with different regions of the central nervous system. In each of the circuits listed below, one or more of the structures has been omitted. Indicate the structure(s) that must be added to complete that circuit.

**361.** Frontal lobe → deep pontine nuclei → cerebellar cortex → _____?_____ → _____?_____ → motor cortex (frontal lobe)

a. Fastigial nucleus → red nucleus
b. Interposed nuclei → red nucleus
c. Dentate nucleus → ventrolateral (VL) nucleus of the thalamus
d. Dentate nucleus → ventral anterior (VA) nucleus of the thalamus
e. Purkinje cell axons → reticular formation of pons

**362.** Red nucleus → inferior olivary nucleus → cerebellar cortex of anterior and posterior lobes → _____?_____ → red nucleus

a. Fastigial nucleus
b. Interposed nuclei
c. Dentate nucleus
d. Purkinje cells of cerebellar hemispheres
e. Vestibular nuclei

**363.** Spinal cord (via dorsal and ventral spinocerebellar tracts) → anterior lobe of cerebellum → _____?_____ → reticular formation and vestibular nuclei → spinal cord

a. Fastigial nucleus
b. Globose nucleus
c. Emboliform nucleus
d. Dentate nucleus
e. Red nucleus

**364.** Based upon your knowledge of the anatomic and neurophysiologic relationships of the anterior lobe of the cerebellum, you would predict that electrical stimulation of the medial vermal aspect of the cerebellar cortex of the anterior lobe will

a. Produce movement of the arms
b. Produce spasticity
c. Cause tonic seizures to occur
d. Modulate extensor muscle tone
e. Have little effect upon muscle tone

**365.** A man presents with a wide-based, ataxic gait during his attempts at walking. He also is unsteady and sways when standing and displays a tendency to fall backward or to either side in a drunken manner. A lesion is most likely located in the

a. Hemispheres of the posterior cerebellar lobe
b. Anterior limb of the internal capsule
c. Dentate nucleus
d. Anterior lobe of the cerebellum
e. Flocculonodular lobe of the cerebellum

# MOTOR SYSTEMS

## *Answers*

**342. The answer is a.** *(Nolte, 3/e, pp 356–358.)* The classic appearance of a patient with a lesion of the cerebellar hemispheres is one in which voluntary and skilled movements are affected. They are uncoordinated and there are errors in the range, force, and direction of movement. The relationships between the cerebellum and the motor regions of the cerebral cortex have been disrupted. Lesions of other regions such as the flocculonodular lobe, vermal region of the anterior cerebellar cortex, or fastigial nucleus produce different symptoms (disturbances of balance, muscle tone, or nystagmus). Although "pure" lesions limited to the ventral spinocerebellar tract have not been reported, it is likely that such a lesion could not account for the symptoms indicated in this question. Information carried by this tract concerns activity of Golgi tendon organs of muscles of the lower limbs.

**343. The answer is d.** *(Nolte, 3/e, pp 312, 315–316.)* An upper motor neuron paralysis occurs following a lesion of the internal capsule. Such a lesion disrupts not only fibers destined for the spinal cord but others that project to parts of the reticular formation and activate inhibitory reticulospinal mechanisms. Loss of such inhibitory input to spinal cord motor neurons then leads to increased levels of excitation of these neurons. The behavioral manifestation of this process is spasticity. Lesions of ventral horn cells produce a flaccid paralysis. Lesions of the postcentral gyrus primarily produce sensory loss, not spasticity. Since the corpus callosum is concerned with interhemispheric transfer of information, a lesion of this bundle will not produce spasticity. A lesion of the substantia nigra will result in Parkinson's disease, which is associated with tremors at rest and rigidity, but not spasticity.

**344. The answer is b.** *(Carpenter, 8/e, pp 252–253, 282–289. Kandel, 3/e, pp 612–613.)* The largest synaptic potentials produced by cortical stimulation would most likely be seen in spinal motor neurons that innervate distal muscles. One of the primary functions of the corticospinal tract is to control the distal muscles of the hands and fingers. Penfield and others constructed a homuncular map from stimulation studies of the cortex. Such studies reveal that the region of cortex associated with the hands and fingers is considerably larger than those regions associated with the proximal musculature. Accordingly, stimulation of the hand region of cortex would activate more fibers than other cortical regions. It is likely that more ventral horn neurons (located in a lateral position) innervate distal musculature than neurons (located in a medial position) innervate proximal musculature. Since the size of the synaptic potential is a function of both the number of fibers that provide a converging input into a given region and the number of cells that discharge in response to that converging input, it is reasonable to conclude that the largest potentials would be observed following stimulation of the cortical regions associated with the distal musculature. Since neurons situated in the motor cortex project their axons to motor horn cells and interneurons but not to sensory neurons of the dorsal horn (although the component of the corticospinal tract that arises from the parietal lobe does project to the dorsal horn), stimulation of the motor cortex could only produce weak potentials at best among sensory neurons in the dorsal horn.

**345. The answer is b.** (*Kandel, 3/e, pp 105–111, 613–623.*) Motor cortex neurons receive information from the muscle to which they project or from a region of skin related to the function of that muscle. The anatomic pathway includes dorsal column–medial lemniscal fibers that terminate in the ventral posterolateral (VPL) nucleus of the thalamus. Fibers from the VPL nucleus then project to the postcentral gyrus. Fibers from a given region of the primary sensory cortex project to the region of primary motor cortex whose projection target in the spinal cord involves the same muscle group (or body part) from which the sensory stimulus originated. All other choices are incorrect. The properties of membrane potentials of neurons in the motor cortex follow the same principles as those found elsewhere in the nervous system; namely, in the resting state, the cell membrane is more permeable to potassium than to sodium. The red nucleus does not have an ascending projection (and, therefore, cannot be reciprocally connected with the motor cortex). Its fibers project, instead, to the spinal cord and lower brainstem. In general, corticospinal fibers that activate alpha motor neurons that innervate a given muscle group will also synapse with gamma motor neurons associated with that same muscle group. Coactivation of both alpha and gamma motor neurons is an important principle because it enables muscle spindles to react to changes in the length of the muscle even during the process of movement of the limb associated with that muscle. The projection to the cerebellum from the motor cortex is disynaptic. Projections from the cerebellum to the motor cortex synapse in the dentate nucleus and the ventrolateral nucleus of the thalamus.

**346. The answer is b.** *(Noback, 5/e, pp 158–162, 245.)* This constellation of deficits, including paralysis of the lower right face, paralysis of right lower limbs, and right deviation of the tongue, requires a lesion located in the left internal capsule. Since the motor fibers from the cortex that supply all three of these regions (i.e., limbs, lower face, and tongue) are all crossed, a lesion of the internal capsule will produce each of these deficits. Also, recall that the tongue will deviate to the side of the lesion when the lesion affects the lower motor neuron (i.e., cranial nerve XII) directly. When it affects the upper motor neuron (i.e., fibers in the internal capsule), inputs into the contralateral nucleus of cranial nerve XII are affected. Thus, the tongue in this instance will deviate to the side opposite the lesion. A lesion of the pontine tegmentum will not affect descending corticospinal or corticomedullary fibers since these fibers are contained in the basilar part of the pons. A lesion of the medulla would be too caudal to affect cortical fibers that terminate on cells of the facial nucleus whose axons innervate muscles of the lower face.

**347. The answer is c.** *(Kandel, 3/e, pp 619–621.)* The premotor areas play an important role in the programming or sequencing of responses that compose complex learned movements. They receive significant inputs for this process from the posterior parietal lobule and in turn signal appropriate neurons in the brainstem and spinal cord (both flexors and extensors). Lesions of the postcentral gyrus produce a somatosensory loss. Lesions of the precentral gyrus produce paralysis. Neither lesions of the prefrontal cortex nor those of the cingulate gyrus have been reported to produce apraxia.

**348. The answer is b.** *(Kandel, 3/e, pp 648–650.)* The neostriatum (i.e., caudate nucleus and putamen) constitutes the principal, if not exclusive, receiving area for afferent fibers to the basal ganglia. The subthalamic nucleus and the substantia nigra share reciprocal connections with the paleostriatum (i.e., globus pallidus) and the neostriatum, respectively. However, these areas receive few, if any, fibers from the cerebral cortex or the centromedian nucleus of the thalamus, which are the major afferent sources to the basal ganglia. Functions of the claustrum are not well understood, but it is believed to be more closely associated with the neocortex than with the basal ganglia.

**349. The answer is e.** *(Kandel, 3/e, pp 652–654.)* The cerebral cortex is a principal source of afferent fibers to the neostriatum and utilizes glutamate as its transmitter, which is excitatory to caudate neurons. Thus, neither gamma-aminobutyric acid (GABA) nor substance P are transmitters from the cortex to the neostriatum; nor is GABA a transmitter released from the nigrostriatal terminals. Projections from the hypothalamus to the caudate nucleus have never been demonstrated and, presumably, do not exist.

**350. The answer is d.** *(Kandel, 3/e, pp 652–654.)* The major transmitter released at terminals of neostriatal and paleostriatal fibers is gamma-aminobutyric acid (GABA). Thus, the output of the basal ganglia is mainly inhibitory. This suggests that thalamic influences upon the cortex are generated through the process of disinhibition whereby neurons of the basal ganglia are inhibited. The presence of glycine in striatal neurons has yet to be demonstrated. Enkephalins are released from terminals of neostriatal-pallidal fibers but not from other efferent neurons of the striatum. Dopamine is released from brainstem and some adjoining hypothalamic neurons but certainly not from striatal neurons. The neostriatum receives cortical inputs that utilize glutamate, but the release of GABA from terminals of striatal efferent fibers has not been demonstrated.

**351. The answer is c.** *(Kandel, 3/e, pp 652–655.)* The basic principle governing how the basal ganglia control motor activity is that they do so by modulating neurons of the motor cortex and premotor areas (of the ipsilateral side) via synaptic connections in the ventrolateral (VL) and ventral anterior (VA) nuclei of the thalamus. One can see from the circuits:

globus pallidus → ventrolateral nucleus → area 4 of cortex
(medial segment)          (VL)

globus pallidus → ventral anterior nucleus → area 6 of cortex
(medial segment)              (VA)

that damage to the basal ganglia on one side of the brain will affect cortical neurons on the same side. This will result in dyskinesia expressed on the contralateral side of the body because the corticospinal tract is crossed. The other possibilities listed in the question are not viable. Projections of the basal ganglia to brainstem nuclei are minimal. The basal ganglia do not project fibers down to the spinal cord nor do they project to the cerebellum.

**352. The answer is c.** (*Kandel, 3/e, pp 634–635.*) The principal source of afferent fibers to the flocculonodular lobe is the vestibular complex, in particular, the inferior and medial vestibular nuclei. For this reason, this lobe of the cerebellum is sometimes referred to as the "vestibulocerebellum." The red nucleus and cerebral cortex project topographically (via relays in the inferior olivary nucleus and deep pontine nuclei, respectively) to the anterior and posterior lobes. Pathways arising from the spinal cord such as the spinocerebellar tract project to the anterior lobe. Other fibers arising from the spinal cord enter the cerebellum through a relay in the inferior olivary nucleus. Such fibers terminate in both anterior and posterior lobes.

**353. The answer is c.** (*Kandel, 3/e, pp 654–657.*) In Huntington's disease, the essential neurochemical change is in the basal ganglia, where there is a significant reduction in the two transmitters acetylcholine and GABA. In particular, there are reduced levels of choline acetyltransferase, glutamic acid decarboxylase, and GABA.

**354. The answer is c.** (*Kandel, 3/e, pp 654–656.*) A lesion of the subthalamic nucleus results in hemiballism, a form of dyskinesia in which the patient displays severe involuntary movements. It is believed to occur as a result of an imbalance in the output signals of the basal ganglia. There is a change in the relationship between efferent pathways associated with the two pallidal segments (i.e., a direct pathway from the medial pallidal segment to the VL and VA nuclei of the thalamus versus an indirect pathway, involving connections between the lateral pallidal segment, subthalamic nucleus, and substantia nigra). Thus, in hemiballism the indirect pathway is disrupted, resulting in a change in the output signals of the pallidum to the thalamus.

**355. The answer is b.** (*Kandel, 3/e, p 654.*) Choreiform movements have generally been associated with damage to the neostriatum (the cortex and the globus pallidus have occasionally been implicated). Normally, there is a balance in what seems to be opposing effects of acetylcholine, dopamine, and GABA in the neostriatum. In this disorder, the levels of acetylcholine and GABA are significantly reduced. This creates an imbalance in which dopamine levels now become (relatively) too high. Accordingly, effective pharmacologic treatment involves the use of dopamine receptor blockers.

**356. The answer is d.** *(Kandel, 3/e, pp 654–657.)* Tardive dyskinesia, a disorder involving involuntary movements of the mouth, face, and tongue, is caused by long-term treatment with antipsychotic drugs that block or decrease dopaminergic synaptic transmission. Such treatment eventually produces a hypersensitivity in dopamine receptors to dopamine. An imbalance is created between dopamine, GABA, and cholinergic systems within the striatum and this is believed to be responsible for the disorder.

**357. The answer is c.** *(Kandel, 3/e, pp 655–656.)* MPTP (1-methyl-4-phenyl-1, 2, 3, 6-tetrahydropyridine) was discovered by accident when drug abusers who were using a synthetic heroin derivative developed signs of Parkinson's disease. It was discovered that their drug included the contaminant MPTP. As a consequence, MPTP has been applied systemically in a number of experimental animals, resulting in significant decreases in dopamine content of the brain due to the loss of dopaminergic neurons in the substantia nigra. These animals also developed symptoms similar to those seen in Parkinson's patients. For these reasons, this drug is currently being used for research purposes in order to develop a better understanding of this disease and to establish possible drug therapies for its treatment and eventual cure.

**358. The answer is a.** *(Noback, 5/e, pp 255–259. Nolte, 3/e, pp 347–350.)* One of the most important features of the anterior lobe of the cerebellum is that it receives major inputs from structures that mediate information concerning muscle spindle and Golgi tendon organ activity (sometimes referred to as "unconscious proprioception"). The pathways that mediate unconscious proprioception include the dorsal and ventral spinocerebellar tracts and the cuneocerebellar tract. Accordingly, the cerebellar anterior lobe is sometimes referred to as the "spinocerebellum." The fastigial and dentate nuclei receive their principal inputs from the cerebellar cortex and their axons project out of the cerebellum. The posterior lobe receives few, if any, inputs from pathways that mediate unconscious proprioception information.

**359. The answer is c.** (*Kandel, 3/e, p 635. Nolte, 3/e, pp 348–349.*) A unique feature of the connections between cerebral cortex and the cerebellum is the somatotopically organized projection from the cerebral cortex largely to the cerebellar hemispheres (some fibers terminate in the vermis). The somatotopic maps are arranged in both anterior and posterior lobes in a manner that has the distal musculature functionally represented in the lateral aspect of the hemispheres while the proximal musculature is represented toward or in the vermal region. Because of this somatotopic arrangement, the lateral hemispheres are concerned with functions associated with detailed movements of the limbs, while more medial regions are concerned with regulation of the proximal musculature (e.g., postural mechanisms).

**360. The answer is d.** (*Kandel, 3/e, p 630.*) The cerebellar glomerulus consists of mossy fiber terminals, Golgi dendrites, axon terminals of Golgi cells, and granule cell dendrites. The flow of information in the glomerulus is as follows: (1) Information reaches the cerebellar cortex through mossy fibers. (2) Axon terminals of mossy fibers terminate upon dendrites of either granule or Golgi cells. (3) Collaterals of parallel fibers (axons of granule cells) may contact dendrites of Golgi cells, whose axons then "feed back" onto the granule cells. (4) Mossy fiber terminals synapse with Golgi cell dendrites, whose axons then make synaptic contact with the granule cell ("feed forward" mechanism). The axons of the granule cells run parallel to the cortex and perpendicular to the orientation of the Purkinje cell dendrites with which they synapse. The circuitry for feedback and feed forward mechanisms is as follows:

Feedback mechanism:
mossy fiber axon terminal → granule cell dendrites → granule cell
axon → Golgi cell → (inhibits) granule cell

Feed forward mechanism:
mossy fiber axon terminal → Golgi cell dendrites → Golgi cell axon → (inhibits)
granule cell

**361–363. The answers are: 361-c, 362-b, 363-a.** (*Kandel, 3/e, pp 632–636.*) For each of these questions, the central point relates to the projection targets of the relevant deep cerebellar nuclei and their relationship to their afferent sources. In Question 361, note that the inputs from the frontal lobe eventually reach the cerebellar cortex (which involves the cerebellar hemispheres of the anterior and posterior lobes to a large extent). Because many of these cerebellar afferents terminate in the lateral aspect of the hemisphere, the return (or feedback) pathway will initially involve Purkinje cell axons that synapse with cells in the dentate nucleus. Fibers of the dentate nucleus then supply the ventrolateral (VL) nucleus of the thalamus, which, in turn, supplies the primary motor cortex. Question 362 concerns the feedback pathways associated with the red nucleus. Inputs to the cerebellum from the red nucleus utilize the inferior olivary nucleus as a relay. These inputs supply the anterior and posterior cerebellar lobes in a topographic manner. Since many of these fibers are distributed to an intermediolateral position within the cerebellar cortex, Purkinje cells from this area supply the interposed (i.e., globose and emboliform) nuclei. The interposed nuclei, in turn, supply the red nucleus via the superior cerebellar peduncle. In Question 363, the issue concerns the relationship of the cerebellum to those spinal cord mechanisms relating to descending fibers of the vestibulospinal and reticulospinal systems. Recall that many of the spinocerebellar fibers are distributed to the medial vermal region of the anterior lobe. Thus, the return flow of information to the spinal cord with respect to the regulation of muscle tension will involve the vestibulospinal and reticulospinal systems. To achieve this objective, the Purkinje cells of the medial (vermal and paravermal) regions of cerebellar cortex project to the fastigial nucleus. The fastigial nucleus, in turn, projects to both the reticular formation and vestibular nuclei, which then complete the feedback circuit by sending their axons down to the spinal cord.

**364. The answer is d.** (*Carpenter, 8/e, pp 490–491. Kandel, 3/e, pp 632–637.*) This experiment was actually carried out many years ago by several investigators. They observed that stimulation of the medial vermal region of the cerebellar cortex could either inhibit or facilitate extensor muscle tone, depending on the precise site of stimulation. It is most likely that stimulation directly affected local populations of Purkinje cells, which then inhibited other local populations of neurons within the fastigial nucleus. Since the fastigial nucleus (as well as the other deep cerebellar nuclei) has excitatory effects upon its target neurons, inhibition or excitation of the fastigial nucleus following local stimulation of the cerebellar cortex would result in either decreased or increased activation of the vestibulospinal system. Thus, such a mechanism could account for the changes of muscle tone seen after stimulation of the anterior vermal region of cortex.

**365. The answer is e.** (*Noback, 5/e, p 261. Nolte, 3/e, pp 356–358.*) Since the flocculonodular lobe receives and integrates inputs from the vestibular system, it is understandable why lesions that disrupt this integrating mechanism for vestibular inputs would result in difficulties in maintaining balance. Indeed, this is a classic feature of lesions of the flocculonodular lobe but is not associated with lesions in the hemispheres of the posterior lobe, anterior limb of the internal capsule, or the dentate nucleus, which are functionally linked to the frontal lobe. Lesions of the anterior lobe also do not affect mechanisms of balance.

# HIGHER FUNCTIONS

## *Questions*

**DIRECTIONS:** The questions below consist of lettered headings followed by a set of numbered items. For each numbered item select the **one** lettered heading with which it is **most** closely associated. Each lettered heading may be used **once, more than once, or not at all.**

### Questions 366–369

Match each description with the correct structure.

a. Ventral anterior (VA) nucleus of thalamus
b. Centromedian (CM) nucleus of thalamus
c. Anterior nucleus of thalamus
d. Ventral posterolateral (VPL) nucleus of thalamus
e. Mediodorsal (MD) nucleus of thalamus
f. Pulvinar
g. Medial geniculate nucleus
h. Habenular complex

**366.** Stimulation of this structure at a frequency of 6 to 12 Hz produces a cortical recruiting response

**367.** This structure receives inputs from limbic structures and the prefrontal cortex

**368.** Axons arising from this region form the stria medullaris

**369.** This structure receives projections from the subicular cortex of hippocampal formation

## Questions 370–373

For each area listed, find the structure whose axons project to it.

a. Pulvinar
b. Mediodorsal thalamic nucleus
c. Lateral geniculate nucleus
d. Medial geniculate nucleus
e. Ventral posterolateral (VPL) thalamic nucleus
f. Ventral posteromedial (VPM) thalamic nucleus
g. Habenular complex
h. Centromedian nucleus

**370.** Face region of the postcentral gyrus

**371.** Leg region of the postcentral gyrus

**372.** Inferior parietal lobule

**373.** Area 17 of the cerebral cortex

## Questions 374–376

Match each description with the appropriate nucleus.

a. Lateral geniculate thalamic nucleus
b. Medial geniculate thalamic nucleus
c. Ventral anterior thalamic nucleus
d. Centromedian thalamic nucleus
e. Mediodorsal thalamic nucleus
f. Anterior thalamic nucleus

**374.** Projection of its axons to the superior temporal gyrus

**375.** Properties of both a specific and a nonspecific thalamic nucleus

**376.** Projection of its axons to the neostriatum

## Questions 377–381

Match each state with the characteristic EEG finding.

a. Alpha waves
b. Beta waves
c. Delta waves
d. Very high-frequency and high-amplitude waves
e. Low-frequency (2 to 4/s), rectangular waves
f. Theta waves
g. Flat EEG
h. Low-voltage, very low-frequency (< 2/s) waves

**377.** Stage 4 of slow-wave sleep

**378.** Alert state

**379.** Grand mal epilepsy

**380.** Focal seizure

**381.** Quiet wakefulness

**DIRECTIONS:**   Each question below contains five suggested responses. Select the **one best** response to each question.

**382.** Vasopressin is released from the posterior pituitary. However, it is synthesized in the

a. Mamillary bodies
b. Lateral hypothalamus
c. Supraoptic hypothalamic nucleus
d. Ventromedial hypothalamic nucleus
e. Posterior hypothalamus

**383.** Which of the following statements concerning temperature regulation is correct?

a. Stimulation of the posterior hypothalamus results in panting, dilation of blood vessels, and suppression of shivering
b. Neurons in the anterior hypothalamus respond to local warming of hypothalamic tissue but not to warming of the skin
c. Stimulation of the anterior hypothalamus may produce constriction of blood vessels and shivering
d. Neurons in the preoptic region and septal area act in concert to intensify increases in body temperature generated by pyrogens
e. Temperature regulation requires the integration of skeletomuscular, endocrine, and autonomic responses

**384.** The supraoptic nucleus is most closely associated with

a. Feeding behavior
b. Temperature regulation
c. Sexual behavior
d. Shortterm memory functions
e. Water balance

**385.** Lesions of the lateral hypothalamus will likely produce

a. Feeding behaviors
b. Drinking behaviors
c. Sexual behaviors
d. Aphagia
e. Hypertension

**386.** A number of investigations have provided strong evidence that the suprachiasmatic nucleus plays an important role in

a. Water intake
b. Food intake
c. Hypertension
d. Circadian rhythms
e. Short-term memory

**387.** The Klüver-Bucy syndrome is typically associated with lesions of the

a. Septal area
b. Amygdala
c. Cingulate gyrus
d. Medial hypothalamus
e. Lateral hypothalamus

**388.** The central nucleus of the amygdala

a. Projects its axons to the medial hypothalamus via the stria terminalis
b. Is a major receiving area for information concerning tertiary auditory and visual signals
c. Has high concentrations of enkephalins, somatostatin, and dopamine
d. Is a primary location of norepinephrine-containing cell bodies in the forebrain
e. Projects axons that directly inhibit spinal motor neurons

**389.** Neurochemical and related theories of schizophrenia postulate that schizophrenia is

a. Basically caused by environmental factors rather than genetic ones
b. Linked to increases in brain dopamine levels
c. Linked to increases in brain serotonin levels
d. Linked to decreases in brain endorphin levels
e. Linked to decreases in brain neuropeptide levels

**390.** While the hippocampal formation has few if any direct (monosynaptic) connections with the lateral hypothalamus, it is known to modulate functions associated with the hypothalamus. The underlying anatomic substrate for such effects is mediated via a synaptic relay in the

a. Cingulate gyrus
b. Habenular nucleus
c. Mediodorsal thalamic nucleus
d. Septal area
e. Bed nucleus of the stria terminalis

**391.** Which of the following constitutes the Papez circuit?

a. Hippocampal formation → mamillary bodies → anterior thalamic nucleus → prefrontal cortex → hippocampal formation
b. Hippocampal formation → septal area → hypothalamus → hippocampal formation
c. Hippocampal formation → mamillary bodies → anterior thalamic nucleus → cingulate gyrus → hippocampal formation
d. Amygdala → hippocampal formation → mamillary bodies → amygdala
e. Prefrontal cortex → hippocampal formation → septal area → medial hypothalamus → prefrontal cortex

## Questions 392–393

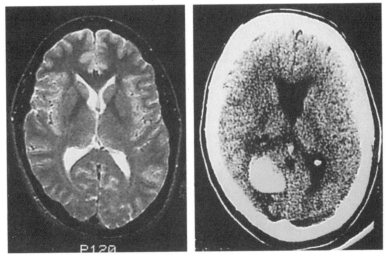

(Courtesy of Alan Zimmer, M.D.)

**392.** The T2-weighted MRI scan on the left side of the figure above is of a normal patient. In the CT scan on the right side, the patient had sustained a right cerebral hemorrhage, indicated by the large white area. It is likely that the cerebrovascular accident produced

a. Right homonymous hemianopsia
b. Left homonymous hemianopsia
c. Loss of intellectual and emotional processes
d. Aphasia
e. Hemiparesis of the right side of the body

**393.** The blood vessel(s) affected in the figure above would most likely be the

a. Anterior cerebral artery
b. Middle cerebral artery
c. Posterior cerebral artery
d. Superior cerebellar artery
e. Striate arteries

## Questions 394–395

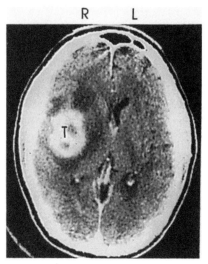

(Courtesy of Alan Zimmer, M.D.)

**394.** The CT scan above reveals that the patient has a glioma (T) on the right side of the brain. It is likely that the patient has sustained

a. An upper motor neuron paralysis of the left side
b. Dyskinesia
c. Intention tremor
d. Upper left quadrantanopia
e. Upper right quadrantanopia

**395.** The tumor in the scan above has most likely damaged the

a. Lentiform nucleus only
b. Internal capsule only
c. Thalamus only
d. Lentiform nucleus and internal capsule
e. Lentiform nucleus, internal capsule, and thalamus

## Questions 396–397

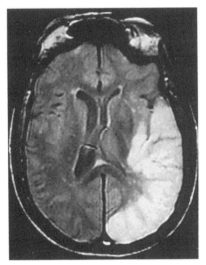

(Courtesy of Alan Zimmer, M.D.)

**396.** The patient whose CT scan is in the figure above sustained an occlusion of a major artery on the left side of the brain. The most prominent deficits will most likely include

a. A right homonymous hemianopsia only
b. Aphasia only
c. A right homonymous hemianopsia coupled with aphasia
d. Marked intellectual deficits
e. Marked intellectual deficits coupled with hemiballism

**397.** The blood vessel occluded in the figure above is the

a. Anterior cerebral artery
b. Middle cerebral artery
c. Posterior cerebral artery
d. Posterior choroidal artery
e. Superior cerebellar artery

## Questions 398–399

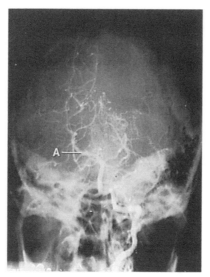

(Courtesy of Alan Zimmer, M.D.)

**398.** The vertebral angiogram in the figure above reveals the effects of a severe motorcycle accident upon a 21-year-old woman. As a result of the accident, she most likely suffers from

a. An upper motor neuron paralysis of the right side of the body
b. A right homonymous hemianopsia
c. A left upper quadrantanopia
d. Aphasia
e. Dyskinesia

**399.** The artery occluded on the left side and labeled in the figure above on the normal side as A is

a. Vertebral
b. Basilar
c. Middle cerebral
d. Anterior cerebral
e. Posterior cerebral

**400.** The MRI scan below reveals a large chromophobe adenoma (T) of the pituitary that impinges on the adjoining brain tissue. This tumor caused a

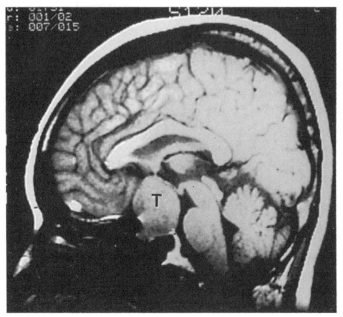

(Courtesy of Alan Zimmer, M.D.)

a. Binasal hemianopsia
b. Bitemporal hemianopsia
c. Loss of the accommodation reflex
d. Loss of the pupillary light reflex
e. Loss of conjugate gaze

# HIGHER FUNCTIONS

## *Answers*

**366–369. The answers are: 366-b, 367-e, 368-h, 369-c.** *(Kandel, 3/e, pp 287–293. Nolte, 3/e, pp 248–264, 397–405.)* Stimulation of the centromedian nucleus (B) at 6 to 12 Hz will produce a recruiting response over widespread areas of the cortex. This response is characterized by a waxing and waning of the signal over an extended period of time. The centromedian nucleus is also a principal source of fibers from the thalamus to the neostriatum. The mediodorsal thalamic nucleus (E) is of considerable importance because of its relationship with the prefrontal cortex with which it maintains reciprocal connections. In addition, it receives significant inputs from other limbic structures such as the amygdala, anterior cingulate gyrus, and septal area. The habenular complex (H), located at the roof of the posterior aspect of the thalamus, receives afferent fibers which reach it by passing through the stria medullaris. The anterior nucleus (C) of the thalamus receives inputs from both mamillary bodies and fornix. The fornix projections arise from the subicular complex of the hippocampal formation.

**370–373. The answers are: 370-f, 371-e, 372-a, 373-c.** *(Nolte, 3/e, pp 248–264.)* The ventral posteromedial (VPM) nucleus (F) is part of the somatosensory pathway for transmission of information to the head region of the cerebral cortex; it thus receives somatosensory inputs from the main sensory and spinal nuclei of the trigeminal complex. The ventral posterolateral (VPL) nucleus of the thalamus (E) is part of an ascending pathway mediating somatosensory information from the body region to the primary somatosensory "body" region of the cerebral cortex. This region is located on the dorsal aspect of the postcentral gyrus and extends over the medial aspect of the cortex. The pulvinar nucleus (A) projects extensively to the inferior parietal lobule and receives inputs from portions of the occipital and temporal lobes associated with integration of visual and auditory signals. The lateral geniculate nucleus (C) is a cortical relay nucleus for the visual system and therefore projects its axons to the primary visual cortex located in area 17.

**374–376. The answers are: 374-b, 375-c, 376-d.** *(Nolte, 3/e, pp 248–264.)* The medial geniculate nucleus (B) projects its axons to the primary auditory receiving areas of the cortex located in areas 41 and 42 of the superior temporal gyrus. The ventral anterior nucleus (C), linked with motor functions of the basal ganglia, receives significant inputs from the globus pallidus and substantia nigra and projects its axons in a diffuse manner to wide areas of the frontal lobe. Moreover, stimulation of this structure has also been reported to have induced recruiting responses in the cortex. Accordingly, the ventral anterior nucleus functions as a nonspecific thalamic nucleus. However, parts of this nucleus also project their axons specifically to the premotor cortex (area 6). The ventral anterior nucleus therefore functions as both a specific and a nonspecific thalamic nucleus. The centromedian nucleus (D) is also a principal source of fibers from the thalamus that innervate the neostriatum (i.e., putamen). Together with the inputs from the cerebral cortex, these two regions (i.e., cerebral cortex and centromedian) constitute the principal afferent sources of the neostriatum.

**377–381. The answers are: 377-c, 378-b, 379-d, 380-e, 381-a.** *(Guyton, 2/e, pp 268–270.)* The EEG response changes during different stages of sleep. In stage 4 of sleep, the EEG frequency becomes very slow with a frequency of approximately 3.5/s or less. This pattern is called a delta wave. When a person is alert, the EEG contains beta waves (B), which are characterized by low voltage and high frequency (> 14 Hz). The EEG typical of grand mal epilepsy has a very high frequency and very high amplitude (D). This is contrasted with the EEG during focal or psychomotor epilepsy in which the waves are low frequency (2 to 4/s) and rectangular in shape (E). Occasionally, a wave of higher frequency is superimposed over the slow waves. During states of quiet wakefulness or drowsiness, the EEG pattern becomes slower (8 to 13 Hz; average amplitude of 50 V) than what is seen during an alert state. This pattern is called an alpha wave (A).

**382. The answer is c.** *(Kandel, 3/e, p 744.)* Certain magnocellular neurons of the hypothalamus synthesize the hormones vasopressin and oxytocin. These include the paraventricular and supraoptic nuclei. The cell bodies of the magnocellular neurons that produce vasopressin are found mostly within the supraoptic nucleus. Vasopressin is important because it makes the membranes of the convoluted tubules and collecting ducts of the kidneys more permeable to water. This results in water conservation.

**383. The answer is e.** *(Kandel, 3/e, pp 752–753.)* The process of temperature regulation requires the integration of autonomic, skeletomuscular, and endocrine responses. For example, dilation of blood vessels of the skin (an autonomic response) facilitates heat loss while constriction of these vessels helps to conserve heat. Panting and shivering (skeletomuscular responses) aid in the processes of heat loss and conservation (heat generation), respectively. Finally, when an organism is exposed to cold for long periods of time, there is an increase in thyroxine release from the anterior pituitary gland, which helps to increase body temperature by increasing metabolism. The classic interpretation of the role of the hypothalamus in temperature regulation has been that the anterior hypothalamus constitutes a heat loss center, while the posterior hypothalamus is a heat conservation center. Although such a generalization is somewhat oversimplified, the general phenomenon has been demonstrated. For example, stimulation of the anterior hypothalamus has been shown to dilate blood vessels and inhibit shivering, and lesions of this region produce hypothermia. Stimulation of the posterior hypothalamus produces heat conservation by constricting blood vessels and causing shivering. Neurons in this region respond to both local warming of hypothalamic tissue as well as to warming of the skin. Neurons in both the septal and preoptic regions constitute antipyretic areas in that they respond to increases in fever by limiting the magnitude of the fever. Activation of these antipyretic regions is thought to occur through a mechanism utilizing the peptide vasopressin. The precise mechanism by which these regions become activated remains unknown.

**384. The answer is e.** *(Kandel, 3/e, p 744.)* The supraoptic nucleus, like the paraventricular nucleus, contains magnocellular neurons that synthesize vasopressin and oxytocin and transport these hormones down their axons to the posterior pituitary. For this reason, the supraoptic nucleus plays a significant role in the regulation of water balance. There is no evidence to support the notion that the supraoptic nucleus has a role in feeding behavior, temperature regulation, sexual behavior, or short-term memory functions.

**385. The answer is d.** *(Kandel, 3/e, p 756.)* Lesions of the lateral hypothalamus are likely to produce aphagia. Feeding behavior is elicited by stimulation of the lateral hypothalamus. Neurons in this region respond to the sight or taste of food. Since drinking is also associated with lateral hypothalamic functions, a lesion of this structure would also disrupt this behavior. Lesions of the lateral hypothalamus do not produce either hypertension or sexual behaviors. The neurons regulating these functions are elsewhere within the hypothalamus.

**386. The answer is d.** *(Kandel, 3/e, pp 758, 801–802.)* Recent studies have demonstrated that the suprachiasmatic nucleus controls the biologic clock of internal circadian rhythms. During the light phase of the light-dark cycle, metabolic activity (measured by $^{14}$C-2-deoxyglucose autoradiography) within the suprachiasmatic nucleus is significantly increased. In contrast, during the dark phase, there is very little metabolic activity.

**387. The answer is b.** *(Kandel, 3/e, p 747.)* In this syndrome, produced experimentally in monkeys and also seen in cats, there is an extreme change in the personality of the animal. Its responses to emotion-laden stimuli are much reduced. It appears very tame. Aggressive tendencies are not evident. It also manifests oral tendencies and displays hypersexuality. This syndrome is the result of lesions of the temporal lobe in which parts of the amygdala are involved. Lesions of other regions such as the hypothalamus, cingulate cortex, or septal area do not produce the Klÿver-Bucy syndrome.

**388. The answer is c.** *(Cooper, 7/e, pp 275–276, 295. Nolte, 3/e, pp 408–412, 418–422.)* One of the most interesting discoveries concerning the amygdala made in recent years is that the central nucleus contains high concentrations of a number of peptides. These include enkephalins and somatostatin in particular. This region also receives large numbers of dopaminergic axon terminals. The central nucleus does not project its axons to the medial hypothalamus. It does not receive auditory or visual signals, nor does it project to the spinal cord, where it could inhibit spinal motor neurons. It receives norepinephrine-containing fibers from the brainstem rather than being a source of this neurotransmitter.

**389. The answer is b.** *(Siegel, 5/e, pp 965–972.)* There have been a variety of neurochemical and related theories of schizophrenia that have evolved over the past three decades. Unfortunately, each of these theories has had its limitation. Nevertheless, one of the more popular theories has been that schizophrenia is linked to increased levels of brain dopamine. The hypothesis suggests that schizophrenia results from overstimulation of the brain by the dopaminergic system. Support for this view comes from the observation that antipsychotic agents are known to block dopamine receptors. Co-twin behavioral and developmental studies have shown that, while environmental factors are certainly important in the ontogeny of schizophrenia, genetic factors are also quite significant in the development of this disease.

Other researchers have suggested that schizophrenia may bear some relationship to decreased levels of serotonin in the brain as evidenced by the hallucinogenic effects of LSD, which binds to serotonin receptors. Other investigations have shown that opioid peptide blockade by naloxone is effective in reducing hallucinations, which suggests that increased levels of endorphins may be linked to this disorder. Investigations involving neuropeptides have indicated that neuropeptides such as cholecystokinin (CCK) is colocalized with dopamine in brain neurons. In this fashion, CCK may function as a neuromodulator for dopamine, in which case increased levels of CCK may be linked with schizophrenia in the same fashion as are increased levels of dopamine.

**390. The answer is d.** *(Nolte, 3/e, pp 266–269, 404–406.)* A major target of efferent fibers from the hippocampal formation is the septal area. Fibers located in the precommissural fornix supply the septal area in an extensive and topographical manner. In turn, the septal area projects significant numbers of fibers to the lateral (and medial) regions of the hypothalamus. In this manner, the septal area serves as a relay for the transmission of signals from the hippocampal formation to the hypothalamus. The hippocampal formation does not project to the habenular nuclei, mediodorsal nucleus, or the bed nucleus of the stria terminalis. Moreover, the cingulate gyrus does not project directly to the hypothalamus.

**391. The answer is c.** *(Noback, 5/e, pp 311–312. Nolte, 3/e, p 406.)* For many years, it was believed that a neural circuit composed of the hippocampal formation → mamillary bodies → anterior thalamic nucleus → cingulate gyrus → hippocampal formation played a major role in the regulation of emotional behavior. More recent studies by a number of investigators have revealed that neither the mamillary bodies nor anterior thalamic nucleus appears to contribute to the regulation of emotional behavior. Instead, it is believed that this circuit may subserve functions more closely related to short-term memory.

**392. The answer is b.** *(Nolte, 3/e, pp 302–304.)* The cerebrovascular accident produced damage of the right primary visual cortex. Therefore, this would result in a homonymous hemianopsia of the left visual fields. Since the damage was confined to the occipital lobe, there would be little effect upon other processes such as speech, motor functions, or intellectual activities.

**393. The answer is c.** (*Nolte, 3/e, pp 76–85.*) The occipital lobe is supplied by the posterior cerebral artery. The calcarine cortex (primary visual cortex) is supplied by a branch of this artery, the calcarine artery. The anterior cerebral artery supplies the medial aspect of the frontal lobe and the anterior-medial aspect of the parietal lobe. The middle cerebral artery supplies the lateral aspect of the frontal and parietal lobes. The superior cerebellar artery supplies the dorsolateral aspect of a portion of the pons and the cerebellum. The striate arteries arise from the anterior and middle cerebral arteries and supply portions of the internal capsule and neostriatum.

**394. The answer is a.** (*Nolte, 3/e, pp 309–311, 319–335.*) The tumor is situated in the lentiform nucleus and internal capsule. Therefore, corticospinal fibers will be affected, causing an upper motor neuron paralysis of the left side. Dyskinesia would not be seen because any effects normally seen in association with damage to the basal ganglia would be masked by the effects of the damage to the internal capsule. Since the cerebellum was not involved, there would be no intention tremor. Neither would there be any visual deficits from this glioma since optic nerve fibers are not involved. The

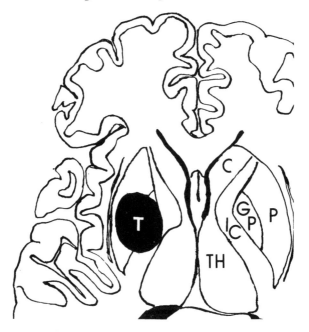

following schematic diagram indicates the approximate extent of the tumor. Labeled are the caudate nucleus (C), the globus pallidus (GP), the internal capsule (IC), the putamen (P), and the tumor (T).

**395. The answer is d.** (*Nolte, 3/e, pp 319–335.*) The tumor clearly involves the lentiform nucleus of the basal ganglia and has expanded to include the internal capsule as well. At the stage when the CT scan was taken, the tumor had not involved the thalamus.

**396. The answer is c.** (*Nolte, 3/e, pp 302–304, 371–388.*) The arterial occlusion involves both the temporal and occipital regions of cortex. Therefore, it would affect Wernicke's area as well as primary visual areas of the occipital lobe. The patient would most likely present with receptive aphasia as well as a right homonymous hemianopsia. The lesion would not likely produce marked intellectual deficits since the prefrontal cortex was spared; nor would it produce hemiballism since there was no damage to the subthalamic nucleus.

**397. The answer is b.** (*Nolte, 3/e, pp 76–85.*) Although the tissue affected involves parietal, temporal, and occipital lobes, the primary artery affected is the middle cerebral artery. The unusual feature of this occlusion is that it appears that the middle cerebral artery extends more caudally than usual. Nevertheless, the middle cerebral artery is the only one of the choices presented that could account for the damage to the temporal and parietal cortices. The anterior cerebral artery supplies the medial aspects of the frontal and parietal lobes; the posterior cerebral artery supplies the occipital cortex (visual areas); the posterior choroidal artery mainly supplies part of the tectum, medial and superior aspects of the thalamus, and the choroid plexus of the third ventricle. The superior cerebellar artery supplies the dorsolateral aspect of a portion of the pons and cerebellum.

**398. The answer is b.** (*Nolte, 3/e, pp 76–85, 302–304.*) An arterial occlusion compromised the blood supply to the occipital lobe on the left side of the brain. Therefore, it would result in a right homonymous hemianopsia with no motor deficits (since no motor regions of the brain are affected).

**399. The answer is e.** (*Nolte, 3/e, pp 76–85, 93–99.*) This vertebral angiogram is an anterior view of the back of the brain. It reveals an occlusion of the left posterior cerebral artery (A). It should be noted that the posterior cerebral arteries are formed from the bifurcation of the basilar artery. Follow the basilar artery caudally (see bottom of the photograph) to the position where it is connected to the vertebral arteries.

**400. The answer is b.** (*Nolte, 3/e, p 303.*) This large pituitary tumor is seen to compress the optic chiasm. Damage to the chiasm affects the crossing fibers of the nasal retina, which convey information from the temporal visual fields. This results in a bitemporal hemianopsia. Since some parts of the optic nerves are spared, pupillary reflexes are preserved. The neuroanatomic substrates for conjugate gaze (i.e., frontal eye fields, pontine gaze center, medial longitudinal fasciculus, and nuclei of cranial nerves III, IV, and VI) are unaffected by the tumor; the mechanism of conjugate gaze remains intact.

# CLINICAL CASES

## Questions

### Clinical Case 1

Sam is a 62-year-old man, previously healthy, who was brought to a neurologist by his daughter because of increasing difficulty walking. His daughter noticed that for the past year, he had difficulty getting out of a chair and took a lot of time to begin to walk. When he did walk, he walked with a slow, shuffling gait. In addition, she had noticed some changes in his face, and that he had been drooling excessively. His signature on checks became progressively smaller from the beginning of his name to the end, and he had developed a new tremor. She brought him in to see if this wasn't just "aging."

The neurologist examined Sam, and noticed immediately that Sam's facial expression was mask-like, with few eye-blinks. When asked to write a sentence, the letters became progressively smaller toward the end of the sentence. His speech was soft and monotonous, and he had a slow, resting "pill-rolling" tremor in both of his hands. He had very little spontaneous movement, and his arms, legs, and trunk were stiff. When the neurologist tried to flex his arm, he felt many catches, similar to a cogwheel. There was no weakness, sensory problems, or abnormalities in his reflexes. When asked to walk, Sam took many tries to rise from his chair. When he finally stood up, his posture was stooped and flexed. His gait was slow, his feet shuffled when he walked, and his arms didn't swing with his steps.

The neurologist told Sam's daughter that she was correct that this wasn't aging, and explained to her all of the details about a new medication that Sam needed to take.

## Questions 401–405

**401.** Damage to which structure in particular causes Sam's problem with movement?

a. Substantia gelatinosa
b. Substantia nigra, pars reticularis
c. Substantia nigra, pars compacta
d. Caudate nucleus
e. Thalamus

**402.** What is the blood supply of the main structure damaged?

a. Lenticulostriate branches of the middle cerebral and anterior cerebral arteries
b. Perforating branches of the basilar and vertebral arteries
c. Anterior choroidal artery and anterior cerebral artery
d. Posteromedial branches of the posterior cerebral and posterior communicating arteries
e. Anterior cerebral and anterior communicating arteries

**403.** What neurotransmitter is deficient?

a. Norepinephrine
b. Glutamate
c. Dopamine
d. Acetylcholine
e. GABA

**404.** Which of the following is a precursor to the deficient neurotransmitter, and can be given as a medication to improve Sam's movement?

a. Tyrosine
b. Choline
c. Acetyl-CoA
d. Tryptamine
e. L-dopa

**405.** The antagonism of which enzyme by drugs will increase the amount of the deficient neurotransmitter?

a. Choline acetyl transferase
b. Monoamine oxidase
c. GABA transaminase
d. Acetylcholinesterase
e. Tyrosine hydroxylase

## Clinical Case 2

Emma is a 64-year-old woman who has had heart disease for many years. While carrying chemicals down the stairs of the dry cleaning shop where she worked, she suddenly lost control of her right leg and arm. She fell down the stairs and was able to stand up with some assistance from a co-worker. When attempting to walk on her own, she had a very unsteady gait, with a tendency to fall to the right side. Her supervisor asked her if she was all right, and noticed that her speech was very slurred when she tried to answer. He called an ambulance to take her to the nearest hospital.

The physician who was called to see Emma in the emergency room noted that her speech was slurred as if she were intoxicated, but the grammar and meaning were intact. Her face appeared symmetric, but when asked to protrude her tongue, it deviated toward the left. She was unable to tell if her right toe was moved up or down by the physician when she closed her eyes, and couldn't feel the buzz of a tuning fork on her right arm and leg. In addition, her right arm and leg were markedly weak. The physician could find no other abnormalities on the remainder of Emma's general medical examination.

## Questions 406–410

**406.** Where in the nervous system has the damage occurred?
a. Right lateral medulla
b. Occipital lobe
c. Left lateral medulla
d. Right cervical spinal cord
e. Left medial medulla

**407.** Where in the nervous system could a lesion occur that causes arm and leg weakness, but spares the face?
a. Right corticospinal tract in the cervical spinal cord
b. Left inferior frontal lobe
c. Left medullary pyramids
d. Occipital lobe
e. Both A and C

**408.** Other than the weakness on her right side, what type of deficit could cause Emma's gait problem and where could a lesion causing this deficit occur?

a. Proprioceptive, left medial lemniscus
b. Sight, left eye
c. Proprioceptive, descending component of the MLF
d. Pain, left spinothalamic tract
e. Proprioceptive, right medial lemniscus

**409.** Deviation of the tongue to the left, away from the right hemiparesis, implies a lesion in which area of the nervous system?

a. Right hypoglossal nucleus
b. Left hypoglossal nucleus
c. Right inferior frontal lobe
d. Left inferior frontal lobe
e. There is no lesion that causes this

**410.** What type of speech problem does Emma have?

a. Broca's aphasia
b. Wernicke's aphasia
c. Mixed aphasia
d. Dysarthria
e. Agnosia

## Clinical Case 3

June is a 65-year-old woman who was previously healthy. One day, while taking a walk in the park, she noticed her right fingers twitching, then her right hand, then her arm and shoulder, followed by a march of twitches down her leg. She did not remember any more than this, because she lost consciousness. An onlooker saw her drop to the ground and deviate her neck backward, while making a high-pitched noise. Then, both of her arms and legs began to jerk for approximately 1 to 2 minutes, then stopped abruptly. She had lost control of her bladder during this event. When the onlooker attempted to speak to June to ask her if she was okay, she was unresponsive. The onlooker called an ambulance, which brought June to the nearest hospital.

A doctor met June at the emergency room entrance, and asked her what had happened. By this time, June was slightly drowsy, but able to answer questions appropriately. Her speech was fluent and grammatically correct. She knew the month, but not the day of the week, or where she was. She moved the left side of her body better than her right, but had too much difficulty following commands for an effective motor examination. The remainder of her examination was normal. The doctor ordered a CT of June's head and drew some blood.

## Questions 411–416

**411.** From which area of the brain did June's seizure begin?
a. Left precentral gyrus
b. Right precentral gyrus
c. Right temporal lobe
d. Left temporal lobe
e. Thalamus

**412.** What could account for June's loss of consciousness following the seizure?
a. Involvement of the reticular activating system
b. Head trauma
c. Bilateral post-ictal suppression
d. Thalamic involvement
e. Brain hemorrhage from the seizure

**413.** The "march" of twitching which June experienced can be explained by

a. Proximity of the body part to the spinal cord
b. Proximity of the body part to the cerebral cortex
c. Somatotopic representation within brainstem
d. Somatotopic representation within the basal ganglia
e. Somatotopic representation within the precentral gyrus

**414.** Which cell type is the predominant cause of the seizure?

a. Basket cell
b. Purkinje cell
c. Stellate cell
d. Schwann cell
e. Pyramidal cell

**415.** A burst of what type of potentials may initiate an epileptic seizure?

a. Inhibitory post-synaptic potentials
b. Membrane potentials
c. Resting potentials
d. Excitatory post-synaptic potentials
e. Nernst potential

**416.** Possible chemical mechanisms that underlie seizure generation include only

a. Na$^+$ channel blockade
b. GABA inhibition
c. Glutamate inhibition
d. Aspartate inhibition
e. GABA agonists

## Clinical Case 4

Julie is a 29-year-old office worker with diabetes, who awoke one morning with the inability to close her left eye, and a left facial droop. Her left eye felt a bit dry, as well. She had run out of sick days, and hoping that the problem would go away, went to work. After several co-workers noticed that her face was drooping, and that she was especially sensitive to loud noises on her left side, they convinced her to go to the nearest emergency room in order to make sure that she did not have a stroke.

She was examined right away in the emergency room, because of her age. The doctor noted immediately that her mouth drooped on the left side. Her left eye was slightly closed. He tested her speech and mental status, which were normal, other than some slight slurring of her speech. Her vision and eye movements were also normal. Sensation and jaw movement were also normal, but when she was asked to wiggle her eyebrows, only the right side of her forehead moved. When asked to close her eyes tightly, and not allow him to open her eyes, her right eye would not open, but her left eye could not oppose the force. She was not able to hold air in her cheeks when asked to hold her breath, and when asked to smile, only the right side of her mouth elevated. She was very sensitive to noise on her left side. When asked to protrude her tongue, it did not deviate to either side, but if she closed her eyes and sugar-water was placed on the left side of the anterior portion of her tongue, she could not identify it. The remainder of her examination was normal. A nurse asked if a head CT should be ordered in order to look for a stroke or tumor, but the doctor said that it was not necessary. He told Julie that he would draw some blood, and give her a medication to take for a while.

## Questions 417–421

**417.** Assuming that the doctor was correct, and that this is not a stroke, where in the nervous system has the damage occurred?

a. Buccinator muscle
b. Trigeminal nerve
c. Facial nerve
d. Glossopharyngeal nerve
e. Hypoglossal nerve

**418.** Julie's facial weakness is characteristic of

a. A muscle lesion
b. A lesion of the internal capsule
c. A superior brainstem lesion
d. An upper motor neuron seventh nerve lesion
e. A lower motor neuron seventh nerve lesion

**419.** Damage to which area may have produced the defect in taste in the anterior two thirds of her tongue?

a. Intermediate nerve
b. Glossopharyngeal nerve
c. Lingual nerve
d. Facial nerve, distal to the chorda tympani nerve
e. Facial nerve, proximal to the chorda tympani nerve

**420.** Assuming that Julie had no prior problems with her ears or cochlear nerve, damage to the nerve supply of which muscle could cause the sensitivity to or distortion of noises?

a. Digastric
b. Platysma
c. Buccinator
d. Geniohyoid
e. Stapedius

**421.** If Julie did not have the loss of taste and noise sensitivity, but did have the inability to move her left eye to the left, which area would now be damaged?

a. The trigeminal and abducens nerves
b. The facial and trigeminal nerves, distal to their exit from the brainstem
c. The facial and abducens nerve nuclei within the pons
d. The facial nerve, distal to the chorda tympani nerve
e. The facial nerve, distal to the geniculate ganglion

## Clinical Case 5

Helen is a 76-year-old woman who has had high blood pressure and diabetes for more than ten years. One day, as she was reaching for a jar of flour in order to make an apple pie, her right side suddenly gave out and she collapsed. While trying to get up from the floor, she noticed that she was unable to move her right arm or leg. Helen attempted to cry for help because she was unable to reach the telephone; however, her speech was slurred and rather unintelligible. She lay on the floor and waited for help to arrive.

Helen's son began to worry about his usually prompt mother when she didn't arrive with her apple pie. After several attempts at telephoning her apartment without an answer, he drove to her apartment and found her lying on the floor. She attempted to tell him what had happened, but her speech was too slurred to comprehend, so assuming his mother had had a stroke, her son called an ambulance to bring her to the nearest emergency room.

A neurology resident was called to see Helen in the emergency room because the physicians there, too, felt she had had a stroke. The resident noted that Helen followed commands very well, and although her speech was very slurred, it was fluent and grammatically correct. The lower two thirds of her face drooped on the right, but when asked to raise her eyebrows, her forehead appeared symmetric. Her tongue pointed to the right side when she was asked to protrude it. Her right arm and leg were severely but equally weak, but her left side had normal strength. She felt a pin and a vibrating tuning fork equally on both sides.

## Questions 422–426

**422.** Where in the central nervous system did Helen's stroke occur?

a. Left precentral gyrus
b. Right precentral gyrus
c. Left basilar pons or left internal capsule
d. Right putamen or globus pallidus
e. Left thalamus

**423.** A computerized tomography (CT) scan revealed a new infarct in the left internal capsule. Which artery was occluded, causing the stroke?

a. Lenticulostriate branches of the middle cerebral artery
b. Posterior cerebral artery
c. Anterior cerebral artery
d. Vertebral artery
e. Posterior choroidal artery

**424.** Damage to which two tracts caused Helen to be weak on her right side?

a. Spinothalamic and corticospinal tracts
b. Spinothalamic and corticobulbar tracts
c. Corticospinal and corticobulbar tracts
d. Corticospinal and spinocerebellar tracts
e. Corticospinal and rubrospinal tracts

**425.** Helen's forehead is spared from the weakness because

a. The forehead is innervated by different fibers originating in the post-central gyrus.
b. There are two cranial nerves innervating the forehead.
c. The forehead is represented bilaterally at the cortical level.
d. The forehead is stronger than the rest of the face.
e. Thalamic regions receiving inputs from the forehead contain few inhibitory neurons.

**426.** How can Helen's speech deficit be classified?

a. Wernicke's aphasia
b. Broca's aphasia
c. Anomia
d. Dysarthria
e. Conduction aphasia

## Clinical Case 6

Audrey is a 45-year-old woman who was brought to her local hospital's emergency room by her husband because of several days of progressive weakness and numbness in her arms and legs. Her symptoms had begun with tingling in her toes, which she assumed to be her feet "falling asleep." However, this feeling did not disappear, and she began to feel numb, first in her toes on both feet, then ascending to her calves and knees. Two days later, Audrey began to feel numb in her fingertips and had difficulty lifting her legs. When she finally was unable to climb the stairs of her house because of her leg weakness, difficulty gripping the banister, and shortness of breath, her husband urged her to go to the emergency room.

The neurologist who examined Audrey in the emergency room noticed that she was short of breath while sitting in bed. He asked the respiratory therapist to measure her vital capacity (the greatest volume of air that can be exhaled from the lungs after a maximal inspiration), and the value for this was far lower than was expected for her age and weight. Her neurologic examination showed that her arms and legs were very weak, so that she had difficulty lifting them against gravity. She was unable to feel a pin or a vibrating tuning fork at all on her legs and below her elbows, but was able to feel the pin on her upper chest. The neurologist could not elicit any reflexes from her ankles or knees. He subsequently advised the emergency room staff that Audrey needed to have a spinal tap, and be admitted to the intensive care unit immediately.

## Questions 427–431

**427.** Where in the nervous system is the damage?
a. Frontal lobe
b. Temporal lobe
c. Peripheral nerves and nerve roots
d. Spinal cord
e. Muscle

**428.** Audrey can't feel a pinprick in certain locations. Which receptor carries this information?

a. Merkel disc
b. Ruffini corpuscle
c. Pacinian corpuscle
d. C and A-delta fibers
e. Meissner

**429.** Which receptor should be activated by the tuning fork?

a. C and A-delta fibers
b. Merkel
c. Pacinian
d. Ruffini
e. Meissner

**430.** The absent reflexes are a sign of a lesion of which portion of the nervous system?

a. The frontal lobe
b. The dorsal horn of the spinal cord or any point distal to this structure
c. Brainstem
d. Cervical corticospinal tract
e. Any point proximal to the upper cervical spinal cord

**431.** Damage to which nervous system structure caused the difficulty breathing?

a. Medullary respiratory center
b. Diencephalon
c. Pons
d. Phrenic nerve innervating the diaphragm
e. Trigeminal nerve

## Clinical Case 7

Lindsey is a 12-year-old girl who has never had medical problems. One day, while in the kitchen with her mother, she told her mother that she felt very frightened all of a sudden, and had a funny feeling in her stomach. Immediately after this, she turned her head to the right, stared persistently, and began to chew. Her mother called her name several times, but Lindsey, who was usually a very obedient child, did not answer. After approximately one minute of staring, Lindsey slowly turned her head back to her mother. Apparently confused, she asked her mother where she was. Over the next 10 to 15 minutes, she became less and less confused, and by the time she was in the car being driven to the pediatrician by her mother, she felt like she was back to normal.

The pediatrician listened to Lindsey's mother's story when they arrived. He examined Lindsey, and could find no abnormalities on general physical examination, or on neurologic examination. The pediatrician told her mother that he would refer Lindsey to a pediatric neurologist for further evaluation, as well as further evaluation for the need for medication.

## Questions 432–436

**432.** What type of problem did Lindsey most likely have?

a.  Attention deficit disorder
b.  Temporary psychosis
c.  Conversion disorder
d.  Epilepsy
e.  Schizophrenia

**433.** From which area of the brain is this problem most likely emanating?

a.  Medulla
b.  Occipital lobe
c.  Temporal lobe
d.  Thalamus
e.  Midbrain

**434.** If the amygdala is involved with this problem, which two major efferent pathways from this structure may be effected?

a. Corticospinal tract and stria terminalis
b. Mamillothalamic tract and stria terminalis
c. Medial forebrain bundle and stria terminalis
d. Ventral amygdalofugal pathway and stria terminalis
e. Corticospinal tract and mamillothalamic tract

**435.** If the hippocampal formation is involved in this problem, which structures may be damaged?

a. Hippocampus, dentate gyrus, and subiculum
b. Hippocampus, amygdala, and subiculum
c. Hippocampus, fornix, and amygdala
d. Hippocampus, fornix, and habenulae
e. Hippocampus, dentate gyrus, and fornix

**436.** If Lindsey develops this problem with a high frequency, what ongoing problem may she eventually develop?

a. Hemiparesis
b. Diminished memory function
c. Diminished sensation
d. Improved attention
e. Dyslexia

## Clinical Case 8

A second-year medical student was asked to see a nursing home patient as a requirement for a Physical Diagnosis course. The patient was a 79-year-old man who was apparently in a coma. The student wasn't certain of how to approach this case, so he asked the patient's wife, who was sitting at the bedside, why this patient was in a coma. The wife replied: "Oh, Paul isn't in a coma. But he did have a stroke." Slightly confused, the student leaned over and asked Paul to open his eyes. He opened his eyes immediately. However, when asked to lift his arm or speak, Paul did nothing. The student than asked Paul's wife if she was certain that his eye opening was not simply a coincidence, and that he really was in a coma, since he was unable to follow any commands.

Paul's wife explained that he was unable to move or speak as a result of his stroke. However, she knew that he was awake, because he could communicate with her by blinking his eyes. The student appeared rather skeptical, so Paul's wife asked her husband to blink once for "yes" and twice for "no." She then asked him if he was at home and he blinked twice. When asked if he were in a nursing home, he blinked once. The student than asked him to move his eyes, and he was able to look in his direction. However, when the student asked him if he could move his arms or legs, he blinked twice. He also blinked twice when asked if he could smile. He did the same when asked if he could feel someone moving his arm. The student thanked Paul and his wife for their time, made notes of his findings, and returned to class.

## Questions 437–441

**437.** Where in the nervous system could a lesion occur that can cause paralysis of the extremities bilaterally, as well as the face, but not of the eyes?

a. High cervical spinal cord bilaterally
b. Bilateral thalamus
c. Bilateral basal ganglia
d. Bilateral pontine tegmentum
e. Bilateral frontal lobe

**438.** An infarct in what vascular distribution could cause this lesion?

a. Anterior spinal artery
b. Vertebral artery
c. Basilar artery
d. Middle cerebral artery
e. Posterior cerebral artery

**439.** Damage to which tracts caused Paul's inability to move his arms and legs?

a. Corticospinal and corticobulbar tracts
b. Spinothalamic tract
c. Tractus solitarius
d. Brachium conjunctivum
e. Superior cerebellar peduncle

**440.** Damage to which tract caused Paul's lack of perception of someone moving his arm?

a. Corticospinal and corticobulbar
b. Middle cerebellar peduncle
c. Spinothalamic tract
d. Rubrospinal tract
e. Medial lemniscus

**441.** What area is spared to preserve consciousness?

a. Deep frontal white matter
b. Pontine reticular formation
c. Temporal lobes
d. Prefrontal cortex
e. Occipital lobe

## Clinical Case 9

Gary is a 35-year-old man who was previously healthy until one day he noticed that his right leg was weak. As the day progressed, he found that he was dragging the leg behind him when he walked, and he finally asked a friend to drive him home from work because he was unable to lift his right foot up enough to place it on the gas pedal. He also noticed that his left leg felt a little bit numb. Finally, his wife convinced him to go to the emergency room of his local hospital.

When Gary arrived at the emergency room, he was having a great deal of difficulty walking. The physician who examined him asked him when this began, and when Gary thought about it in more depth, he realized that perhaps this had started slowly several days before, and he had ignored the symptoms. Gary's language function, cranial nerves, and motor and sensory examinations of his arms were within normal limits. When the physician examined Gary's right leg, it was markedly weak, with very brisk reflexes in the knee and ankle. Vibration and position sense in the right leg were absent. Pain and temperature testing were normal in the right leg, but these sensations were absent on the left leg and abdomen to the level of his umbilicus. Reflexes in the left leg were normal, but when the physician scratched the lateral portion of the plantar surface on the bottom side of Gary's right foot, the big toe moved up. The remainder of Gary's examination was normal.

### Questions 442–446

**442.** What area of the nervous system is damaged?

a. Brainstem
b. Cervical spinal cord
c. Thoracic spinal cord
d. Frontal lobe
e. Peripheral nerves

**443.** Damage to which tract could give Gary the loss of vibration and position sense on the right side?

a. Right fasciculus cuneatus
b. Right fasciculus gracilis
c. Left fasciculus cuneatus
d. Left fasciculus gracilis
e. Right Lissauer's tract

**444.** Gary's loss of left-sided pain and temperature sensation could be due to damage of which tract?

a. Right fasciculus cuneatus
b. Right fasciculus gracilis
c. Right spinothalamic tract
d. Left spinothalamic tract
e. Left corticospinal tract

**445.** Why is Gary's right leg weak?

a. There is muscle damage in the right leg
b. There is damage in his left frontal lobe
c. There is damage to the right corticospinal tract
d. The dorsal root is damaged
e. There is damage to the right femoral nerve

**446.** The upward movement of Gary's toe when the plantar surface of his foot was scratched is indicative of a lesion in which portion of the nervous system?

a. Upper motor neuron
b. Lower motor neuron
c. Peripheral nerves
d. Muscles
e. Sural nerve

## Clinical Case 10

Jane is a 75-year-old woman who has taken medication for high blood pressure and high cholesterol for the past ten years. One morning, upon awakening, she attempted to get up from her bed, only to find that she had difficulty walking, but didn't know why. When she tried to walk, her left leg collapsed beneath her. Jane couldn't understand why she was having so much difficulty waking, because she felt fine. Thinking that perhaps something was wrong, she edged her way across the floor to her telephone and promptly called for an ambulance. Jane hadn't noticed until now that her speech was slightly slurred. She was taken to the nearest emergency room for an evaluation.

Upon arriving in the emergency room, the staff noted that her face drooped on the left and that she persistently looked to her right side, and called a neurologist to see Jane. The neurologist tested Jane's language functions by asking her to name objects, repeat sentences, and write sentences, and thought that all of these tests were normal. Her speech was mildly slurred, and she had a right gaze preference. She would not cross the midline with her eyes when asked to look to the left, but instead, immediately returned her eyes to their right-sided gaze. When asked to raise her left hand, she raised her right hand. The neurologist asked Jane if her left hand belonged to her and she replied "no, it's yours." When asked to fill in the numbers of a clock, Jane put numbers 1 through 12 on the right side of the clock. When asked to bisect a line, she placed the perpendicular line on the right side. She did not blink to hand waving in the temporal visual field of her left eye, and the nasal visual field of her right eye. Other cranial nerves were normal, except for a left facial droop which spared the forehead. Her left arm and leg were markedly weak and the muscle tone was flaccid (floppy). All reflexes were depressed on the left side and normal on the right. The neurologist thought that all sensory modalities were depressed on the left side. The neurologist ordered a CT scan of Jane's head, and admitted her to the hospital for further work-up and treatment.

## Questions 447–451

**447.** What kind of neurologic deficits does Jane have?

a. Left hemiparesis, hemineglect, left homonymous hemianopsia, left hemisensory loss
b. Left hemiparesis, right superior quadrantanopsia
c. Left hemiparesis, left hemisensory loss, hemineglect, left superior quadrantanopsia
d. Left hemisensory loss, hemineglect, bitemporal hemianopsia
e. Left hemisensory loss, hemineglect, left superior quadrantanopsia

**448.** Where in the nervous system has the damage occurred?

a. Left temporal and parietal lobes
b. Right frontal and temporal lobe
c. Right frontal and parietal lobes
d. Left frontal and parietal lobes
e. Left occipital lobe

**449.** If this damage was caused by a stroke, which artery became occluded?

a. Right anterior cerebral artery
b. Left anterior cerebral artery
c. Right posterior cerebral artery
d. Right middle cerebral artery
e. Left middle cerebral artery

**450.** Damage to which fibers caused Jane's inability to blink in response to the hand waving in her left temporal visual field?

a. Left facial nerve
b. Right oculomotor nerve
c. Left optic nerve
d. Optic chiasm
e. Right optic radiations

**451.** Damage to which specific area caused Jane's inability to notice the left side of her body?

a. Left anterior frontal cortex
b. Right anterior frontal cortex
c. Right posterior frontal cortex
d. Right posterior parietal cortex
e. Right anterior parietal cortex

## Clinical Case 11

Herb, a 62-year-old man, who has smoked two packs of cigarettes per day for 35 years, was suffering from a chronic cough that was attributed to a smoking habit by his physician. One day, Herb noticed that his right eyelid drooped slightly, and that his right pupil was smaller than the left. He also noticed that the inner side of his right hand was numb, and that he had begun to drop things from his right hand. He had no other symptoms. Herb consulted his physician who directed him to a neurologist.

The neurologist noted that although the right pupil was smaller than the left, it was still reactive to light. Although Herb's right eyelid drooped slightly, he could close his eyes tightly when asked to do so. The neurologist noted that Herb did not sweat on the right side of his face. He was unable to feel a pinprick on the inner surface of his right hand, and his right triceps and hand muscles were weak.

## Questions 452–456

**452.** Where in the nervous system has damage occurred?

a. Left oculomotor nerve
b. Right oculomotor nerve
c. Nucleus of Edinger-Westphal
d. Sympathetic fibers coursing from the hypothalamus to the intermediolateral cell column
e. Parasympathetic fibers coursing from the nucleus of Edinger-Westphal

**453.** Herb's small pupil is due to

a. Unopposed action of muscles with parasympathetic innervation
b. Unopposed action of muscles with sympathetic innervation
c. Both sympathetic and parasympathetic damage
d. A lesion in the nucleus of the third nerve
e. A lesion in distal branches of the trochlear nerve

**454.** Why was Herb able to close his eye tightly, despite a drooping eyelid?

a. The facial nerve does not innervate muscles mediating eye closure
b. The facial nerve is only partially affected
c. The facial nerve is unaffected by this lesion
d. The trigeminal nerve compensates for eye closure
e. This lesion only affects involuntary eye closure

**455.** Which pair of neurotransmitters is involved in the pathway which has been damaged?

a.  Substance P and acetylcholine
b.  Norepinephrine and epinephrine
c.  5-HT and GABA
d.  GABA and acetylcholine
e.  Acetylcholine and norepinephrine

**456.** Damage to which fibers caused the numbness and weakness of his hand?

a.  Ipsilateral cerebral peduncle
b.  Corticospinal tract
c.  Cervical spinal roots entering the brachial plexus
d.  Basilar artery
e.  Median nerve

## Clinical Case 12

Morris is a 79-year-old man who was brought to the emergency room (ER) because his family was worried that he suddenly was not using his right arm and leg, and seemed to have a simultaneous behavior change. He was unable to write a reminder note to himself, even with his left hand, and he put his shoes on the wrong feet. A neurologist was called to the ER to examine the patient. A loud bruit (pronounced *bru-e*; a rumbling sound) was heard with a stethoscope over the left carotid artery in his neck. When asked to show the neurologist his left hand, he pointed to his right hand, since it could not move. The neurologist asked him to add numbers, and he was unable to do this, despite having spent his life as a bookkeeper. Morris was unable to name the fingers on either hand, and he could not form any semblance of a letter, using his left hand. His eyes did not blink when the neurologist waved his hands close to Morris's eyes in the left temporal and right nasal visual fields. The right lower two thirds of his face drooped. There was some asymmetry of his reflexes between the right and left sides, and there was a positive Babinski response of his right toe.

### Questions 457–461

**457.** Where in the central nervous system is the damage?

a.  Right frontal and parietal lobes
b.  Left frontal and parietal lobes
c.  Right frontal lobe
d.  Left frontal lobe
e.  Right temporal lobe

**458.** Assuming that Morris had a stroke, which artery has become occluded?

a.  Left anterior cerebral
b.  Right anterior cerebral
c.  Right middle cerebral
d.  Left middle cerebral
e.  Left posterior cerebral

**459.** Damage to which area of the brain caused Morris's inability to move his right side?

a. Right precentral gyrus
b. Left precentral gyrus
c. Right angular gyrus
d. left angular gyrus
e. Left supramarginal gyrus

**460.** Damage to which region caused Morris's inability to tell right from left, and his inability to write, even with his nondominant hand?

a. Left parietal
b. Left frontal
c. Right frontal
d. Left temporal
e. Right temporal

**461.** Damage to which structure caused the visual defect?

a. Right optic nerve
b. Left optic nerve
c. Optic chiasm
d. Right optic radiations
e. Left optic radiations

## Clinical Case 13

John is a 57-year-old man who has always been a very heavy drinker, often consuming two pints of whiskey per day, for many years. Upon the urging of his wife, he decided to seek medical attention for help with problems with his gait, which has steadily worsened over the past several months. He noticed that he now needed to stand with his feet far apart in order to maintain his balance, and "waddled" when he walked.

The doctor who evaluated him tested his memory and speech careful-ly, as well as his cranial nerves, and was unable to find any deficits. There was no weakness, sensory loss, or abnormalities in his reflexes. When asked to touch the doctor's finger, then his nose, John missed his nose slightly, but rapidly corrected the movement on both sides. When asked to slide his right heel down his left shin, his heel slid sideways and clumsily across the bone until it reached his ankle. The response with the left heel was similar. When asked to walk, John walked with his feet very far apart. If he attempted to walk in a tandem fashion, with one heel in front of the other toe, he began to fall, and the doctor needed to catch him. The doctor ordered an MRI (magnetic resonance imaging) of John's head.

### Questions 462–467

**462.** What term could one use for John's gait?

a. Stiff
b. Festinating
c. Ataxic
d. Spastic
e. Shuffling

**463.** A gait problem of this type could be caused by lesions in which sys-tem(s)?

a. Cerebellar tracts only
b. Posterior columns only
c. Corticospinal tracts
d. Both the cerebellar and posterior column systems
e. Spinothalamic system

**464.** Where in the brain would a neurologist expect to visualize the lesion on a magnetic resonance image scan (MRI scan)?

a.  Red nucleus
b.  Cerebellar vermis
c.  Substantia nigra
d.  Internal capsule
e.  Basilar pons

**465.** The region of the affected area is associated with which functional division of the cerebellum?

a.  Cerebrocerebellum
b.  Spinocerebellum
c.  Dentate nucleus
d.  Brachium conjunctivum
e.  Brachium pontis

**466.** To which deep nucleus does the damaged region project?

a.  Globose
b.  Dentate
c.  Fastigial
d.  Vestibular
e.  Emboliform

**467.** Which cell type most likely sustained the most damage from John's alcohol consumption?

a.  Schwann cell
b.  Pyramidal cell
c.  Stellate cell
d.  Anterior horn cell
e.  Purkinje cell

## Clinical Case 14

Bob is a 75-year-old male college graduate who was brought to a neurologist by his family because he was having problems with his gait, suffered from urinary incontinence for the past six months, and recently began to have problems with his short-term memory and paying his bills. The gait problem mainly manifested itself as difficulty in climbing stairs and frequent falls. Bob had no past medical history other than a subarachnoid hemorrhage resulting from a ruptured cerebral aneurysm many years earlier.

When the neurologist examined Bob, she found that he could not remember three objects five minutes after they were shown to him, even when he was prompted. He was unable to figure out how many quarters were in $1.75, and spelled the word "world" incorrectly. A grasp reflex (squeezing the examiner's hand as a reflex reaction to stroking of the palm) was present. Although his motor strength was full in all of his extremities, when asked to walk, he took many steps in the same place without moving forward, then started to fall. His cranial nerve, sensory, and cerebellar examinations were normal.

## Questions 468–471

**468.** Bob has a grasp reflex and dementia. A lesion in which region can cause this deficit?
a.  Occipital lobe
b.  Frontal lobe
c.  Medulla
d.  Thalamus
e.  Pons

**469.** You are asked to evaluate Bob with the neurologist. The nurse in the office asks if you would like to order a CT (computerized tomography) scan, and you request one. The CT scan shows that all the ventricles are dilated, especially the frontal horns of the lateral ventricles, without any evidence of obstruction by a tumor. What would be a possible mechanism underlying the enlargement of the ventricles?

a. Decreased CSF absorption
b. Low blood pressure
c. Decreased CNS blood flow
d. Decreased intracranial pressure
e. High blood pressure

**470.** If there is diminished CSF absorption, where does the blockage occur?

a. Pyramidal cells
b. Renshaw cells
c. Arachnoid villi
d. Purkinje cells
e. Sagittal sinus

**471.** Where would the greatest damage be done by the expanding ventricles?

a. Thalamus
b. Brainstem
c. Pituitary gland
d. Parietal cortex
e. Deep frontal white matter (corona radiata)

**Clinical Case 15**
Joe is a 75-year-old man who is right-handed and was told in the past by his internist that he had an irregular heartbeat. Unfortunately, Joe decided that he didn't wish to learn anything further about this condition, so he didn't return to this physician and it remained untreated. One morning, he awoke to find that his face drooped on the right side, and that he couldn't move his right arm or right leg. When he tried to call an ambulance for help, he had a great deal of difficulty communicating with the operator because his speech was slurred, non-fluent, and missing some pronouns. The call was traced by the police, and an ambulance arrived at his house and brought him to an emergency room.

A neurologist was called to see Joe in the emergency room. When he listened to Joe's heart, he detected an irregular heartbeat. It was very difficult to understand Joe's speech, because it was halting, with a tendency to repeat the same phrases over and over. He had a great deal of difficulty repeating specific sentences given to him by the neurologist, but he was able to follow simple commands such as: "touch your right ear with your left hand." His mouth drooped on the right when he attempted to smile, but his forehead remained symmetric when he wrinkled it. He couldn't move his right arm at all, but was able to wiggle his right leg a little bit.

**Questions 472–476**

**472.** What kind of language problem does Joe have?
a.  Dysarthria
b.  Wernicke's aphasia
c.  Broca's aphasia
d.  Alexia
e.  Pure word deafness

**473.** Which area of the brain is damaged?
a.  Internal capsule and thalamus
b.  Right occipital lobe
c.  Pontine reticular formation
d.  Corpus callosum
e.  Left pre-central gyrus and Broca's area

**474.** Which artery was blocked when the event occurred?

a. Anterior cerebral artery
b. Posterior cerebral artery
c. Anterior inferior cerebellar artery
d. Middle cerebral artery
e. Basilar artery

**475.** Which term best describes Joe's facial weakness?

a. Peripheral VII nerve
b. Central VII nerve
c. XII nerve
d. V nerve
e. Oculomotor nerve weakness

**476.** With which hand does Joe most likely write?

a. Right
b. Left
c. Ambidextrous (both)

## Clinical Case 16

Susan is a 32-year-old woman who recently stopped taking her birth control pills in order to become pregnant. However, after several months, her menstrual period failed to resume. Prior to beginning the birth control pills several years before, she had been having normal cycles. She also noticed headaches, which had been increasing in severity over the past several months. Recently, she became aware of difficulty with her peripheral vision. Thinking that she might be pregnant, she sought the attention of her gynecologist.

Her doctor ran a pregnancy test, which was negative. She told her that there may be another cause of the absence of her menstrual cycle, and she sent Susan's blood for levels of various hormones. When Susan returned to find out the results of the tests, her gynecologist told her that the level of the hormone prolactin was high. Susan remembered her headaches and visual symptoms, and informed her doctor, who promptly referred her to a neurologist.

The neurologist listened to Susan's story, and examined her. She found only that Susan was unable to see fingers in the temporal fields (lateral half of each visual field) of both of her eyes. The remainder of her neurologic exam was normal. The neurologist told Susan that she would like to order an MRI (magnetic resonance imaging) test of her head, in order to find out why she had the headaches, visual problem, and high prolactin levels.

## Questions 477–481

**477.** A tumor in which area could cause a high prolactin level?

a. Adenohypophysis
b. Neurohypophysis
c. Amygdala
d. Hippocampus
e. Adrenal gland

**478.** What type of neurologic visual loss can cause a loss of peripheral vision?

a. Central scotoma
b. Superior quadrantanopsia
c. Bitemporal hemianopsia
d. Homonymous hemianopsia
e. Papilledema

**479.** A lesion adjacent to which structure caused Susan's visual problem?

a. Optic nerve
b. Optic radiations
c. Retina
d. Optic chiasm
e. Lateral geniculate nucleus

**480.** Which hypothalamic nucleus regulates prolactin secretion?

a. Suprachiasmatic nucleus
b. Preoptic nucleus
c. Paraventricular nucleus
d. Supraoptic nucleus
e. Arcuate nucleus

**481.** Which neurotransmitter system regulates prolactin secretion?

a. Tuberoinfundibular dopaminergic system
b. Nigrostriatal dopaminergic system
c. Mesolimbic dopaminergic system
d. Mesocortical dopaminergic system
e. Mesostriatal dopaminergic system

## Clinical Case 17

Mike is a 35-year-old man who had optic neuritis (an inflammation of the optic nerve causing blurred vision) several years before. He was told that he had a 50 percent chance of eventually developing multiple sclerosis, a degenerative disease of the CNS white matter. One day, he noticed that he had double vision and felt weak on his right side. Although he noted that the symptoms were becoming steadily worse throughout the day, he attributed this to stress from his job as a stockbroker, and in order to relax, he decided to take a drive in his car. While he was driving, his vision became steadily worse. As he was about to pull over to the side of the road, he saw two trees on the right side of the road. Uncertain which was the actual image, he attempted to place his right foot on the break pedal. Mike suddenly realized that he was unable to lift his right leg, and his car collided with the tree. A pedestrian on the side of the road called EMS, and Mike was brought to a nearby emergency room.

A neurologist was called to see Mike because the emergency room physicians thought he may have had a stroke, despite his young age. The neurologist spoke to Mike, then examined him. He found that his left eye was deviated to the left and down. When he attempted to look to his right, his right eye moved normally, but his left eye was unable to move further to the right than the midline. His left pupil was dilated and did not contract to light from a penlight. His left eyelid drooped, and he had difficulty raising it. In addition, the right side of his mouth remained motionless when he attempted to smile, but his forehead was symmetric when he raised his eyebrows. Mike's right arm and leg were markedly weak. The neurologist told Mike that he wasn't certain that this was necessarily a stroke, but admitted him to the hospital for observation and tests.

## Questions 482–486

**482.** A lesion in which nerve caused Mike's double vision?

a.  Optic nerve
b.  Oculomotor nerve
c.  Cervical sympathetic fibers
d.  Trochlear nerve
e.  Abducens nerve

**483.** Damage to nerves innervating which eye muscles cause Mike's eye to be deviated towards the left side and down?

a. Superior rectus, superior oblique, inferior rectus, inferior oblique
b. Superior rectus, inferior rectus, inferior oblique, lateral rectus
c. Superior rectus, inferior rectus, inferior oblique, medial rectus
d. Lateral rectus, superior oblique, medial rectus, inferior rectus
e. Lateral rectus, superior oblique, inferior oblique, medial rectus

**484.** Where in the nervous system did the damage occur?

a. Left frontal lobe
b. Right frontal lobe
c. Left eye
d. Cervical spinal cord
e. Midbrain

**485.** Damage to which fibers caused the enlarged, unreactive left pupil?

a. Medial longitudinal fasciculus
b. Frontal or pontine eye fields
c. Edinger-Westphal nucleus or preganglionic parasympathetic fibers
d. Trochlear nerve
e. Cervical sympathetic fibers

**486.** Damage to which area caused Mike's weakness?

a. Left precentral gyrus
b. Right precentral gyrus
c. Left cervical spinal cord
d. Right cervical spinal cord
e. Left cerebral peduncle

## Clinical Case 18

Louise is an 86-year-old woman who has had difficulty with high blood pressure, high cholesterol, diabetes, strokes, and blood clots in her legs for many years. One day, her grandson arrived at her apartment in a senior citizen center for his weekly visit, only to find her lying unconscious on the floor. He immediately called an ambulance to bring her to the nearest emergency room.

The paramedics in the ambulance gave Louise some medications, including glucose, but she did not awaken. She was brought to the nearest emergency room, where a physician was called to evaluate her. She was breathing on her own and had a pulse, but could not be aroused to any stimulus. Her arms and legs were stiff, and would not move in response to a painful stimulus. Her eyes moved in response to moving her head. Finally, in response to a very loud shout and pinch on the arm, she briefly opened her eyes, however she immediately shut them again. Further attempts to arouse Louise were unsuccessful. She was taken for a CT scan of her head, and then brought to an intensive care unit.

### Questions 487–491

**487.** An acute stroke in which portion of the central nervous system could cause this situation?

a. Right frontal lobe
b. Left frontal lobe
c. Right temporal lobe
d. Pons and midbrain
e. Right occipital lobe

**488.** What is the cause of the stiffness in Louise's arms and legs?

a. Infarction of the corticospinal tracts bilaterally in the pons
b. Damage to the basal ganglia
c. Infarction of the precentral gyrus
d. Infarction of the internal capsules bilaterally
e. Thalamic infarction

**489.** Infarction of which artery may cause this picture?

a. Anterior cerebral artery
b. Middle cerebral artery
c. Anterior choroidal artery
d. Basilar artery
e. Lenticulostriate branches of the middle cerebral artery

**490.** If the stroke occurred in the brainstem, which region is most likely affected?

a. Facial nerve nucleus
b. Trochlear nerve nucleus
c. reticular formation
d. Trigeminal system
e. Medial longitudinal fasciculus

**491.** What are the main monoaminergic systems of the region infarcted?

a. Dopamine only
b. Norepinephrine only
c. Serotonin only
d. Melatonin only
e. Norepinephrine and serotonin

## Clinical Case 19

Norma is a 75-year-old woman who had a stroke several months ago, manifested by numbness on her right side, including her arm, face, trunk, and leg. The numbness had improved somewhat over time, but did not completely disappear. One day, she noticed that brushing her right arm against a door was very painful. Thinking that perhaps this was "in her mind," she tried touching the right arm with her left hand, and this, too, was painful. Fearful that she may be having another stroke, she went immediately to see her neurologist at her local hospital.

Norma's neurologist examined her and found that sensation for a pin, temperature, and vibration were diminished on the entire right side of her body. The degree of sensory loss was unchanged from an examination several months before. However, she had a large amount of discomfort with any type of stimulus, accompanied by some emotional disturbance. The discomfort was far out of proportion to the degree of the stimulus; for instance, a light touch to her right arm would engender a scream similar to that elicited by a knife. The remainder of her examination was normal.

The neurologist told Norma that he didn't think that she had had a new stroke, but would order a head CT to be sure that there was no tumor or bleeding. In addition, he told her that if the head CT showed nothing new, that she could begin a new medication which would help with the pain.

### Questions 492–496

**492.** What is the most likely location of the old stroke?
a. Right precentral gyrus
b. Left precentral gyrus
c. Right ventral thalamus
d. Left ventral thalamus
e. Left cerebral peduncle

**493.** Which two nuclei mediating sensation of the arms, face, legs, and trunk may have sustained damage from the original stroke?

a. Lateral and medial geniculate nuclei of the thalamus
b. Ventral posterior lateral and ventral posterior medial nuclei of the thalamus
c. Putamen and globus pallidus
d. Caudate and putamen
e. Anterior and lateral dorsal nuclei of the thalamus

**494.** Which pathway mediating pain is the afferent input into the infarcted area?

a. Tractus gracilis
b. Tractus cuneatus
c. Spinocerebellar tract
d. Spinothalamic tract
e. Corticospinal tract

**495.** Surgical stimulation of various regions of the central nervous system has been shown to alleviate pain. What is the location of one of these areas producing analgesia?

a. Anterior nucleus of the thalamus
b. Caudate nucleus
c. Anterior horn of the spinal cord
d. Globus pallidus
e. Periaqueductal gray

**496.** Neurotransmitters implicated in pain modulation, which may be the targets of pain-alleviating drugs, include

a. Aspartate
b. Glutamate
c. Epinephrine
d. Dopamine and norepinephrine
e. Opiates and serotonin

## Clinical Case 20

A 17-year-old high school football player presented to a neurology clinic because his mother thought that he may have acquired neck problems during a game. A month before, he had sustained a concussion from a blow to his head from another player. Shortly after, she noted that he intermittently tilted his head to the side. When asked what was the matter, he simply said that sometimes he had double vision, and that the images were situated on top of each other vertically, making it difficult to go down stairs. When examined, there was no neck pain or limitation of motion. He tended to keep his head tilted to the right side. When asked to follow the doctor's finger with his head in a straight position, his left eye would not move downward when his eyes were turned to the right, and tended to remain slightly deviated toward the left. At this point, he stated that he had double vision, and felt better if his head was tilted to the right. The remainder of his eye movements, as well as the remainder of his exam was normal.

## Questions 497–501

**497.** Where has the damage occurred?

a. The oculomotor nerve
b. The abducens nerve
c. The trochlear nerve
d. The trigeminal nerve
e. The facial nerve

**498.** Which muscle is weakened?

a. Superior rectus
b. Inferior rectus
c. Lateral rectus
d. Superior oblique
e. Inferior oblique

**499.** From which portion of the brainstem has the damaged nerve emerged?

a. Right ventral midbrain
b. Right dorsal midbrain
c. Left ventral midbrain
d. Left dorsal midbrain
e. Left ventral pons

**500.** What is the action of the weak muscle?

a. Outward and upward rotation of the eye
b. Outward and downward rotation of the eye
c. Inward and upward rotation of the eye
d. Inward and downward rotation of the eye
e. Deviation of the eye laterally

**501.** How could the head trauma have caused the double vision?

a. Direct damage to the eye
b. Damage to the occipital lobes
c. Damage to the midbrain
d. Damage to the pons
e. Damage to the cranial nerve peripherally

# CLINICAL CASES

## *Answers*

**401. The answer is c.** (*Kandel, 3/e, pp 654–656.*) Sam has Parkinson's disease, a degenerative condition caused by progressive loss of dopaminergic cells in the substantia nigra pars compacta. This is an area that controls the speed and spontaneity of movement, so damage to this area can produce deficits that include: a slow, shuffling gait with a tendency to move progressively faster ("festinating" gait), problems with maintaining size in handwriting, with a tendency to write with small letters (micrographia), masklike facial expression with a paucity of eye-blinks, and difficulty getting out of a chair. Other problems include a soft, monotonous voice, muscle rigidity (lead-pipe rigidity), a tremor at rest which is "pill-rolling," and a combination of a tremor and rigidity, especially in the arms, which, when flexion is attempted, elicits a "cogwheeling" property. Failure to swallow with a normal frequency makes drooling a problem. Dementia (senility) is also a problem with Parkinson's patients, especially later in the course of the disease.

**402. The answer is d.** (*Kandel, 3/e, p 1042.*) The blood supply to the substantia nigra arises from the posterior circulation, specifically the posteromedial branches of the posterior cerebral artery and branches of the posterior communicating artery. The lenticulostriate branches of the middle cerebral artery supply other portions of the basal ganglia, such as the striatum and the globus pallidus. The anterior choroidal artery also supplies some of the telencephalic nuclei of the basal ganglia.

**403. The answer is c.** (*Kandel, 3/e, pp 654–656.*) The majority of cells that are lost in this disease are dopaminergic cells in the substantia nigra, pars compacta. Only the pars compacta region of the substantia nigra contains dopaminergic neurons.

**404. The answer is e.** (*Kandel, 3/e, p 655.*) Medications are currently available to lessen the symptoms of Parkinson's disease. Some of these medications contain various concentrations of L-dopa, an immediate precursor to dopamine. Dopamine itself doesn't cross the blood-brain barrier, so it cannot be directly replaced.

**405. The answer is b.** *(Adams, 6/e, p 1074.)* Medications that antagonize the breakdown of catecholamines by monoamine oxidase can increase the amount of dopamine available for the remaining cells in the substantia nigra.

**406. The answer is e.** *(Adams, 6/e, p 799.)* Emma has had a stroke resulting from occlusion of medial branches of the left vertebral artery, presumably secondary to atherosclerosis (i.e., cholesterol deposits within the artery which eventually occlude it). The resulting syndrome is called the *medial medullary syndrome*, because the affected structures are located in the medial portion of the medulla. These structures include: the pyramids, the medial lemniscus, the medial longitudinal fasciculus, and the nucleus of the hypoglossal nerve and its outflow tract. Emma's symptoms result from damage to the above structures, and may have been caused by the same process (atherosclerosis) that resulted in her heart disease.

**407. The answer is e.** *(Adams, 6/e, p 799.)* The weakness of her right side was caused by damage to the medullary pyramid on the left side. Her face was spared because fibers supplying the face exited above the level of infarct. However, a lesion in the corticospinal tract of the cervical spinal cord above C5 could cause arm and leg weakness, and spare the face, because facial fibers exit in the rostral medulla. A lesion in the inferior portion of the precentral gyrus of the left frontal lobe would cause right-sided weakness, but would include the face, because this area is represented more inferiorly than are the extremities.

**408. The answer is a.** *(Adams, 6/e, p 799.)* Her unsteady gait was a result of the weakness of her right side, but may also have been the result of the loss of position and vibration sense on that side from damage to the medial lemniscus (as demonstrated by the inability to identify the position of her toe with her eyes closed, and the inability to feel the vibrations of a tuning fork). Without position sense, walking becomes unsteady because it is necessary to feel the position of one's feet on the floor during normal gait. Damage to both the medial lemniscus and pyramids at this level cause problems on the contralateral side because this lesion is located rostral to the level where both of these fiber bundles cross to the opposite side of the brain. Damage to the descending component of the MLF could only affect head and neck reflexes, but not gait. Gait is also unaffected by pain inputs.

**409. The answer is b.** (*Kandel, 3/e, pp 684–685. Adams, 6/e, p 1383.*) Deviation of the tongue occurs because fibers from the hypoglossal nucleus innervate the genioglossus muscle on the ipsilateral side of the tongue. This muscle normally protrudes the tongue toward the contralateral side. Therefore, if one side is weak, the tongue will deviate toward the side ipsilateral to the lesion when protruded. A lesion in the precentral gyrus causes protrusion of the tongue toward the side contralateral to the lesion because it is rostral to the crossing of fibers into the hypoglossal nucleus.

**410. The answer is d.** (*Adams, 6/e, p 1383.*) Her speech was dysarthric (slurred) because her tongue was weak on the left side. The physician saw this during the exam when her tongue deviated to the left when protruded. Since the weakness of the tongue is a purely motor problem—rather than an effect manifest by a lesion to higher centers in the cortex that mediate the structure and function of speech—the grammar, content, and meaning of Emma's speech remained intact, as would be expected with an aphasia or agnosia.

**411. The answer is a.** (*Kandel, 3/e, p 785.*) June had a seizure, which began focally on the left motor strip (the left precentral gyrus), moved up the motor strip, then secondarily generalized, or spread, throughout the cortex. The phenomenon whereby there is twitching of an extremity that spreads to other areas on that extremity or other areas of the body is called a "Jacksonian march." This phenomenon is named for Hughlings Jackson, a neurosurgeon who was instrumental in mapping out the cerebral cortex and describing the somatotopic organization of the cortex of the prefrontal gyrus called a homunculus (meaning "little man"). Observing patients with a Jacksonian march helped him to identify areas represented at each location of the motor strip.

**412. The answer is c.** (*Kandel, 3/e, p 789.*) Very often, there is inhibition following a seizure, which accounts for drowsiness or a "post-ictal state" after the seizure has finished. Sometimes, epileptic discharges spread to other areas of the cortex, recruiting contiguous areas of cortex through callosal, commissural, and sometimes thalamic circuits to eventually involve a large area of the cortex, causing the movements of the entire body. This occurs with a generalized seizure. If the cortex of both hemispheres become involved, there may be impairment or loss of consciousness. The cells (often pyramidal cells) in the cortex can generate a seizure through high-frequency, synchronous discharges in large groups. If the seizure begins focally, as this one did, there may be a "Todd's paralysis," as June had, where there is transient paralysis of the involved motor area during the post-ictal period.

**413. The answer is e.** *(Kandel, 3/e, p 785.)* There is somatotopic organization of the motor strip (see answer for Question 412), and cortical neurons are included among the most likely to generate seizures, making this area the most likely to cause such a pattern.

**414. The answer is e.** *(Kandel, 3/e, pp 782–787.)* The pyramidal cell is a cell in the cortex that uses glutamate, an excitatory neurotransmitter, whereas most other types of cortical neurons use GABA, an inhibitory neurotransmitter. The spike, one identifying feature of an epileptic seizure seen on electroencephalogram recorded on the scalp, is initiated by a depolarization shift, which is thought to be generated by excitatory post-synaptic potentials.

**415. The answer is d.** *(Kandel, 3/e, p 787.)* Excitatory post-synaptic potentials are considered to be an initiating cellular event for a seizure (see answer for Question 414). In order to become a seizure, however, the cellular discharges require enhancement and synchronization.

**416. The answer is b.** *(Kandel, 3/e, pp 787–789.)* Since seizure generation requires excitation, or a loss of inhibition, the only correct choice is the inhibition of GABA, an inhibitory neurotransmitter. All the other choices cause inhibition only. Many new anticonvulsant medications are currently being designed to either enhance GABA activity or inhibit the excitatory neurotransmitter, glutamate.

**417. The answer is c.** *(Wilson-Pauwels, p 88. Adam, pp 1376–1377.)* This is an example of Bell's palsy, or damage to the facial nerve distal to its nucleus in the pons. The motor weakness is lower motor neuron because of the involvement of the upper one third of the face (this has bilateral inner-vation within the central nervous system). The loss of taste on the anterior two thirds of the tongue and the hyperacusis (sensitivity to noise) point to damage distal to the brainstem because these are functions whose nerves join the facial nerve distal to its exit from the pons. This type of palsy may be caused by a virus, and is more common among people with diabetes.

**418. The answer is e.** *(Wilson-Pauwels, p 88.)* This type of facial paralysis, involving the upper one third of the facial muscles, is characteristic of a lower motor neuron facial nerve lesion. Since there is bilateral innervation within the central nervous system, from the prefrontal gyrus bilaterally, until their synapse at the facial nerve nucleus, all upper motor neuron fa-cial weakness spares the forehead.

**419. The answer is e.** *(Wilson-Pauwels, p 94. Kandel, 3/e, p 691.)* Since there is motor weakness of the face, and the chorda tympani nerve, which subserves taste, joins the facial nerve, it is likely that the lesion exists prox-imal to where the chorda tympani joins the facial nerve. A lesion in the lin-gual nerve (a branch of the trigeminal) would result in a loss of taste, as well, but would also result in a loss of sensation to the face, not motor weak-ness. If the lesion occurred distal to the chorda tympani nerve, taste would have been spared.

**420. The answer is e.** *(Wilson-Pauwels, p 86. Kandel, 3/e, p 691. Adams, p 1376. Noback, p 236.)* The facial nerve sends a branch to the stapedius mus-cle distal to the geniculate ganglion, but proximal to the chorda tympani nerve. Lesions proximal to this branch will cause weakness of the stapedius muscle. Contraction of this muscle normally serves as a mechanism for dampening the motion of the ossicles, thus lowering the amount of stimu-lation reaching the Organ of Corti. If this muscle is paralyzed, hyperacusis (increased acuity) as well as hypersensitivity to low tones will occur.

**421. The answer is c.** *(Wilson-Pauwels, p 87.)* Since the genu of the facial nerve is in close proximity to the nucleus of the abducens nerve, the pons is a likely location for this particular type of combination of findings. Since the damage to the facial nerve has occurred distal to the facial nerve nu-cleus, a lower motor neuron facial palsy is present. The lack of hyperacu-sis and the presence of normal taste imply that the lesion is proximal to the geniculate ganglion. Therefore, the lesion must be between the facial nerve nucleus and the geniculate ganglion, and the location in the pons is the most likely choice. If this clinical picture is present, then an infarct or tumor in the pons must be suspected, and in this case, an imaging study would be more appropriate.

**422. The answer is c.** *(Kandel, 3/e, p 543.)* A CT scan of Helen's head was done in the emergency room, which showed a new infarct or stroke in the genu and anterior portion of the posterior limb of the left internal capsule. This is the region of the internal capsule through which most of the fibers of the corticospinal and corticobulbar tracts pass in a somatotopically organized fashion before entering the brainstem. Because most of these fibers pass through a very small region, a small infarct can cause deficits in a wide distribution of areas. In this case, Helen has weakness on her face and tongue, causing her slurred speech, in addition to weakness of her arm and leg. In addition, since somatosensory fibers destined for the postcentral gyrus occupy a position in the internal capsule caudal to the corticospinal tract fibers, these fibers are spared and Helen has no sensory deficits. The only other area in the central nervous system that can cause a pure motor hemiparesis is the basilar pons, an area through which corticospinal and corticobulbar fibers also run. The vascular supply of this region consists of perforators from the basilar artery, which are small and subject to atherosclerotic disease.

**423. The answer is a.** *(Kandel, 3/e, p 1042.)* The internal capsule is supplied primarily by the lenticulostriate branches of the middle cerebral artery. In addition, portions of the posterior limb of the internal capsule are supplied by the anterior choroidal artery, a branch of the internal carotid artery. Both the lateral striate branches and the anterior choroidal artery are small branches of larger arteries, and are more susceptible to damage (atherosclerosis) from high blood pressure and diabetes than the larger vessels.

**424. The answer is c.** *(Kandel, 3/e, p 543.)* The corticospinal and corticobulbar tracts contain motor fibers originating in the precentral gyrus, mediating voluntary motor function of the face, arms, legs, and trunk. They pass through the internal capsule to the crus cerebri in the midbrain. The spinothalamic tract is a sensory tract, and could not cause the observed deficits. The rubrospinal tract only affects the spinal cord.

**425. The answer is c.** *(Wilson-Pauwels, p 86.)* Helen's forehead is unaffected by the lesion because the forehead is bilaterally represented on the cortex, so the right side retains innervation despite a lesion in the left internal capsule. Motor fibers from each side pass into the internal capsule ipsilaterally, so a lesion in the internal capsule will not effect the forehead. This type of finding is called a "central seventh nerve lesion," because it represents a lesion in the CNS superior to the level of the seventh nerve nucleus, where the fibers from both sides of the forehead coalesce.

**426. The answer is d.** *(Adams, 6/e, p 1383.)* Dysarthria is slurred speech, occurring from lesions affecting innervation of the tongue, lips, and palate. We are given evidence that her tongue is weak in that it points to the right. The interruption of fibers traveling to the hypoglossal nerve from the left side eventually innervate the right genioglossus muscle, which pulls the tongue to the left. Dysarthria is a motor phenomenon, unlike aphasia, which is a disruption of language. Language is primarily generated in the cerebral cortex; so, because the lesion spares the cortex, there were no signs of aphasia.

**427. The answer is c.** *(Adams, 6/e, pp 43–48, 1312–1318.)* This patient does not have an upper motor neuron lesion (spinal cord or above) because of the absent reflexes and ascending paralysis bilaterally involving all of the extremities. Lesions in the brain almost always give unilateral findings, and spinal cord lesions give a distinct level. The damage cannot be in the muscle, because the patient has sensory involvement as well. This case is an example of Guillain-Barre syndrome (GBS), or an inflammatory disease of peripheral nerve resulting from demyelination. Inflammatory cells are found within the nerves, as well as segmental demyelination and some degree of Wallerian degeneration. This damage can cause an ascending paralysis and sensory loss, affecting the arms, face, and legs. The cerebrospinal fluid often has a high protein level, making a spinal tap a useful test for the diagnosis of GBS. Nerve conduction studies are also helpful in making the diagnosis. Most neurologists believe GBS to be an immunologic reaction directed against peripheral nerve, and some patients have a history of some type of infection prior to developing GBS. However, a clear-cut cause is rarely found. Despite a known cause, most patients recover from GBS, although the speed of recovery varies. Treatment is currently available (administration of gamma globulin), and, if instituted early in the course of the disease, decrease in the length of the illness is possible.

**428. The answer is d.** *(Kandel, 3/e, p 386.)* Pain is mediated by C and A-delta fibers in the skin.

**429. The answer is c.** *(Kandel, 3/e, p 368.)* Pacinian corpuscles best mediate vibration.

**430. The answer is b.** *(Adams, 6/e, pp 43–48.)* The reflexes are lost because the lower motor neurons affected by this process are unable to participate in the reflex arc necessary for a knee or ankle jerk to take place. These lower motor neurons originate with stretch receptors in the tendons. Answers A, C, D, and E are all examples of upper motor neuron lesions, usually characterized by hyperactive reflexes.

**431.  The answer is d.** *(Adams, 6/e, pp 43–48.)* This is an example of a lower motor neuron problem. Answers A, B, and C are upper motor neuron structures. The trigeminal nerve is a cranial nerve, which mediates sensation on the face and the muscles of mastication. Loss of diaphragmatic function causes respiratory distress.

**432. The answer is d.** *(Adams, 6/e, pp 321–322.)* This is an example of a complex partial seizure, most likely originating in the temporal lobe. A seizure is a paroxysmal derangement of the central nervous system due to rhythmic, synchronous discharges from cerebral neurons, causing changes in consciousness, sensation and/or behavior. Complex partial seizures often start with a warning or "aura." Since limbic structures are often involved, the seizure can include emotions, feelings of deja-vu or jamais-vu, or gastrointestinal sensations. Because olfactory pathways end in the temporal lobe, patients may experience "smells" as well. The seizure itself involves impairment of consciousness of some form, often manifested as staring, in addition to various stereotyped, automatic behaviors called *automatisms.* The latter may be manifested as chewing, repetitive swallowing, hand gestures, or vocalizations. These usually occur during the seizure, but may occur after it. After the seizure ends (the seizures usually last 1 to 2 minutes), the patient is often in a confused or postictal state for several minutes, or even up to several hours. Occasionally, a patient may manifest aggressive behavior while in the postictal state. Unless a structural lesion, such as a tumor, is present, the physical examination is usually normal. Verification of the diagnosis of epilepsy is done with the help of an electroencephalogram, or EEG, which records potential differences of summed cortical action potentials over the scalp of a patient. Often, an epileptic spike, or sharp wave, is seen over the area from which the seizures arise. Epilepsy patients usually also have a CT scan or MRI (magnetic resonance imaging) to make certain that there is no structural lesion causing the seizures.

**433. The answer is c.** *(Adams, 6/e, pp 321–322.)* Seizures similar to this one often begin with abnormal neuronal discharges in temporal lobe structures, which include the amygdala or hippocampus. These structures tend to have a lower threshold for this type of activity than other structures in the brain.

**434. The answer is d.** *(Kandel, 3/e, p 737.)* The major descending pathways from the amygdala are the stria terminalis and the ventral amygdalofugal pathway. The medial forebrain bundle is a major pathway of the lateral hypothalamus. The mamillothalamic and corticospinal tracts do not involve the amygdala.

**435. The answer is a.** *(Kandel, 3/e, p 737.)* The hippocampal formation includes the hippocampus, the dentate gyrus, and the subiculum. All of the other structures listed are within the limbic system, but do not lie within the hippocampal formation.

**436. The answer is b.** *(Kandel, 3/e, p 830.)* Since memory is a function mediated by the limbic system, a structure most likely involved in the generation of these seizures, it is possible that Lindsey will have memory problems in the future if she has frequent seizures. Early studies of patients who have undergone resection of portions of one or both temporal lobes have demonstrated the presence of memory deficits.

**437. The answer is d.** *(Kandel, 3/e, p 729.)* This is an example of the "locked-in syndrome," or pseudocoma, caused by an infarction of the pontine tegmentum. Because the tracts mediating movement of the limbs and face run through this region, the patient is unable to move the face, as well as both arms and legs. Consciousness and eye movements are preserved.

**438. The answer is c.** *(Kandel, 3/e, p 729.)* The pontine tegmentum is mainly supplied by the basilar artery. Complete occlusion of this artery causes deficits on both sides, since this artery supplies both sides of the pons.

**439. The answer is a.** *(Kandel, 3/e, p 729.)* Basilar artery occlusion causes damage to the basilar pons, where the corticospinal and corticobulbar tracts run. These tracts contain motor fibers mediating movement of the limb and face, respectively. This results in complete paralysis to both sides of the body and the face. None of the tracts in the other choices mediate conscious movement.

**440. The answer is e.** *(Adams, 6/e, p 805.)* Sensory loss, including loss of proprioception (feeling the movement of a limb) also occurs as a result of damage to the medial lemniscus bilaterally. This tract contains fibers from the dorsal columns, and also runs through the pontine tegmentum.

**441. The answer is b.** *(Adams, 6/e, p 802.)* Patients with the "locked-in syndrome" are often mistaken for comatose patients due to their inability to move or speak. If the lesion spares the reticular formation, an area mediating consciousness in the pons, the patient will remain alert.

**442. The answer is c.** *(Kandel, 3/e, p 718.)* Gary has a spinal cord syndrome called Brown-Sequard syndrome, or hemisection of the spinal cord. The lesion is not at the cervical level because motor functions of the upper limbs were considered normal. The examiner can pinpoint the location of the lesion by using the "sensory level" or level at which the loss of pain and temperature begin, by remembering that the lesion affects fibers that have entered the spinal cord 1 to 2 levels below it, and then cross to the contralateral side. Therefore, a loss of sensory function at $T_{10}$ level indicates a lesion at $T_8$ or $T_9$ level. A level at which motor deficits begin can be helpful as well, but in lesions of the thoracic spinal cord, muscles innervated by thoracic nerves are difficult to test. The examiner still expects weakness in the lower extremities, and this helps to make the diagnosis. The Brown-Sequard syndrome may occur as a result of different types of tumors or infections of the spinal cord.

**443. The answer is b.** *(Kandel, 3/e, p 718.)* Because one half of the spinal cord is damaged, the dorsal columns are damaged, and the patient will have loss of proprioception and vibration ipsilateral to and below the level of the lesion. The loss must be ipsilateral because fibers mediating this type of sensation cross above the level of the lesion. The fasciculus gracilis carries fibers originating from the sacral, lumbar, and lower thoracic levels, and the fasciculus carries those from the upper thoracic and cervical levels. Lissauer's tract carries pain and temperature fibers via the dorsal root entry zone. The Brown-Sequard syndrome may occur as a result of different types of tumors or infections of the spinal cord.

**444. The answer is c.** *(Kandel, 3/e, p 718.)* The spinothalamic tract carries fibers mediating pain and temperature. The primary pain fibers enter the spinal cord and pass 1 to 2 segments in the zone of Lissauer before making synapse with neurons that form the lateral spinothalamic tract. Fibers of the lateral spinothalamic tract then cross to the contralateral side 1 to 2 segments above or before where the primary afferent fibers have entered the cord. Accordingly, pain and temperature are lost below the lesion on the contralateral side. The cuneate and gracile fasciculi mediate proprioception and vibration, and the corticospinal tract mediates voluntary motor function.

**445. The answer is c.** *(Kandel, 3/e, p 718.)* The corticospinal tract mediates voluntary motor function. The fibers cross in the medullary pyramids; thus lesions below this structure cause ipsilateral weakness. The reflexes are brisk, since in an upper motor neuron lesion there is a loss of inhibition to spinal reflexes. Muscle, dorsal root, and femoral nerve damage are all examples of lesions distal to the spinal cord. A frontal lobe lesion would not cause a sensory or motor level, and would probably cause problems more proximally, such as slurred speech.

**446. The answer is a.** *(Kandel, 3/e, p 718.)* A positive Babinski sign or dorsiflexion of the great toe when the lateral portion of the plantar surface of the foot is scratched is a sign of corticospinal tract dysfunction, a tract consisting of upper motor neurons. Peripheral nerve (including the sural nerve) lesions are lower motor neuron lesions.

**447. The answer is a.** *(Kandel, 3/e, pp 831–832. Adams, 6/e, pp 456–457.)* Jane is not only unable to move her left side (hemiparesis), but ignores its existence (anosognosia or the syndrome of hemineglect, see below). Even though she neglects her left side, the blink reflex should still be intact if she only neglects the side. Therefore, a visual field deficit called a homonymous hemianopsia is present on the left side (see figure), in which the left temporal and right nasal fields are damaged. There may also be some degree of primary sensory loss, which can be difficult to evaluate when a patient neglects the same side.

**448. The answer is c.** (*Adams, 6/e, pp 443–446, 456–457.*) Jane's deficits result from lesions of the posterior frontal cortex, as well as from some contribution of corticospinal tract fibers to the parietal lobe and deeper motor cortical structures. In addition, the neglect and hemisensory loss result from damage to the parietal cortex. The homonymous hemianopsia results from damage to the deep portion of the parietal lobe where the optic radiations pass to the superior and inferior banks of the visual cortex, causing the visual field defect.

**449. The answer is d.** (*Kandel, 3/e, p 1045.*) The posterior frontal lobe, as well as parietal lobe, are supplied by the middle cerebral artery. Areas supplied by this artery, such as primary and supplementary motor areas, and the primary and secondary somatosensory cortices may be effected. As a result, the patient may have left-sided weakness, upper motor neuron facial weakness that spares the forehead, and hemisensory loss.

**450. The answer is e.** (*Kandel, 3/e, p 1045.*) If the lesion is deep enough, the patient may have a visual field cut called a homonymous hemianopsia, where fibers traveling from the optic chiasm to the occipital cortex within the optic radiations are interrupted, and the patient doesn't see the left temporal and the right nasal visual field. It is common for patients with neglect not to notice the areas of blindness because they ignore the left side. Patients with this problem are usually advised not to drive a car.

**451. The answer is d.** (*Kandel, 3/e, pp 831–832. Adams, 6/e, pp 456–457.*) Jane's problem is an example of the syndrome of hemi-neglect, which arises from a lesion of the posterior parietal lobe. This area is essential for spatial organization. If this area, usually on the nondominant (right) side, is no longer functioning, the patient will live in a world which consists solely of a right side. Patients with a syndrome of hemi-neglect will look only to the right side (if the lesion is on the right), and when asked to look to the left, often will not cross the midline with their eyes. Especially when the lesion is acute, these patients will not acknowledge any person or objects on their left side, and it is not unusual for a patient to complain of losing her glasses when they are on a table on her left side. Since these patients see only the right side of everything, they will put all of the numbers of a clock on the right side of the clock, and will bisect a line on its right side. In addition, they will only comb the right side of their hair, dress the right side of their bodies, and shave the right side of their faces. When confronted with a left-sided entity, such as a left arm, they will often ignore the question, or may even go as far as claiming it belongs to someone else. In resolving lesions where the patient now has sensation and acknowledgment on the left side, she may still display extinction to double simultaneous stimuli, where if both sides are touched simultaneously, the patient feels the touch only on the right side and "extinguishes" the stimulus on the left. However, it is important to remember that neglect can resemble weakness because the patient won't move the left side.

**452. The answer is d.** *(Adams, 6/e, p 280, 538.)* Herb's drooping eyelid, small pupil, and lack of sweating on the right side are examples of Horner's syndrome. This is caused by the interruption of sympathetic fibers anywhere along their course from the hypothalamus and brainstem to the intermediolateral cell column in the upper thoracic levels of the spinal cord where neurons, supplying sympathetic innervation to the pupil, the levator palpebrae superioris muscle of the eyelid, and sweat glands of the face, are located.

**453. The answer is a.** *(Adams, 6/e, p 280, 538.)* Interruption of this sympathetic innervation will result in the drooping of the upper eyelid (ptosis), pupillary constriction (miosis; due to unopposed action of the parasympathetic innervation of the circular muscles of the iris) and lack of sweating on the face. Parasympathetic or oculomotor damage causes pupillary dilation, rather than constriction.

**454. The answer is c.** *(Kandel, 3/e, p 692.)* Herb could close his eyes tightly because this function is mediated by the seventh nerve, which is not damaged by this lesion.

**455. The answer is e.** *(Kandel, 3/e, pp 762–770. Adams, 6/e, p 280.)* Preganglionic sympathetic neurons are predominantly cholinergic and postganglionic sympathetic neurons are predominantly noradrenergic. Horner syndrome may be caused by either a preganglionic or postganglionic lesion. The location may be determined by the use of eyedrops specifically targeted at a particular neurotransmitter.

**456. The answer is c.** (*Adams, 6/e, p 538.*) One cause of interruption of the sympathetic fibers is a tumor of the apex (top portion) of the lung called a Pancoast tumor. Because the apex of the lung is in close proximity to the spine, a Pancoast tumor may compress the upper thoracic spinal cord where the sympathetic fibers exit from it. Compression of the adjacent spinal nerves between C8 and T2, entering the brachial plexus, also interrupts the nerve supply to the hand and triceps muscle, causing numbness and weakness in these areas. Pancoast tumors do not often cause respiratory symptoms early on in their course because they are located far from the mainstem bronchi. Because these tumors have this unique location, the neurological abnormalities often pre-date the respiratory problems. The neurologist suspected that Herb may have Pancoast tumor in the lung because of his long history of smoking.

**457. The answer is b.** (*Adams, 6/e, pp 443–445, 453–459.*) This case is an example of a lesion of the left (usually dominant) parietal lobe, most often in the angular gyrus, with some involvement of the precentral gyrus in the posterior frontal lobe. There is contralateral upper motor neuron weakness (with a positive Babinski sign), as well as several cortical sensory defects, specifically, right-left confusion, agraphia (inability to write, independent of motor weakness), acalculia (inability to calculate), and finger agnosia (inability to designate the fingers). The latter four elements are sometimes referred to as Gerstmann syndrome by neurologists, and all represent spatial discriminatory functions of the parietal lobe (often the dominant parietal lobe, which is usually the left). The parietal lobe also subserves other visual-spatial functions such as construction of complex drawings. There are other locations within the central nervous system where upper motor neuron weakness can occur; however, the combination with parietal lobe signs can only occur in this location. If the damage was slightly more extensive, it may have involved Broca's area, causing aphasia.

**458. The answer is d.** (*Kandel, 3/e, pp 1041–1043.*) The artery serving this region (both posterior frontal and parietal lobes) is the right middle cerebral artery, which originates at the Circle of Willis. Because it continues in a nearly straight line from the internal carotid artery, it is a common route for small emboli formed from blood clots in the internal carotid artery. The bruit noted over the right common carotid artery in this patient is most likely a result of a thrombus (clot) which occludes part of the lumen of the artery. These emboli can occlude the middle cerebral artery because it is considerably smaller than the internal carotid artery. Since the middle cerebral artery has many branches through which an embolus may travel, but the territory of this stroke is large, it is likely that the embolus lodged in a more proximal location in this case.

**459. The answer is b.** *(Kandel, 3/e, pp 1043–1045.)* Morris's leg weakness includes a positive Babinski sign, which is an upper motor neuron sign. Although this type of weakness may occur in several locations in the central nervous system, the combination with the cortical parietal signs can only occur in the left precentral gyrus if there is to be one lesion.

**460. The answer is a.** *(Adams, 6/e, pp 443–445, 453–459.)* These deficits are visual-spatial in nature, and are characteristic of damage to the dominant parietal lobe (see also answer for Question 451).

**461. The answer is e.** *(Kandel, 3/e, p 1045.)* The visual defect that Morris experiences is a homonymous hemianopsia, resulting from damage to the optic radiations traveling from the lateral geniculate nucleus to the visual cortex in the occipital lobe. These split, so that inferior images are carried through the parietal lobe, and superior images through the temporal lobes, but in large infarcts, the defect is more likely to involve more fibers of this tract. Since the optic radiations carry representations of the ipsilateral temporal field and the contralateral nasal field (only the nasal field fibers cross), this defect is noted clinically as the inability to detect objects in the regions described. Often the patient will only notice bumping into objects on the side ipsilateral to the stroke, since turning of the eyes can compensate for the nasal field defect.

**462. The answer is c.** *(Kandel, 3/e, p 684. Adams, 6/e, p 89.)* An ataxic gait is an unsteady gait. Gaits due to motor weakness or spasticity tend to involve circling of the weak leg (circumduction), and festinating or shuffling gaits, often due to Parkinsonism or disease of the basal ganglia involve a stooped posture with shuffling of the feet and very small steps.

**463. The answer is d.** *(Kandel, 3/e, p 684. Adams, 6/e, pp 89, 118.)* An ataxic gait may result from motor incoordination due to cerebellar disease, or from lack of proprioception in the lower extremities due to disease in the posterior column system (gait becomes unsteady when a patient is unable to detect the location of his/her feet). Degeneration of both systems may occur due to alcoholism, although in this case, we are told that John does not have any sensory deficits when this modality is tested in isolation.

**464. The answer is b.** *(Adams, 6/e, pp 1156–1158.)* This is an example of alcoholic cerebellar degeneration. It is caused by degeneration (probably through nutritional deficiency) of neurons in the cerebellar cortex, particularly of the Purkinje cells, and is usually restricted to anterior and superior parts of the vermis, as well as anterior portions of the anterior lobes. For this reason, most of the deficits in this syndrome involve midline structures such as the trunk, which is represented most in the vermis. Trunk instability usually causes problems with gait. In addition, because the cerebellar homunculus represents the legs in the anterior portion of the anterior lobe, the legs are affected more than the arms. Loss of volume within the vermis of the cerebellum is readily visualized, especially on an MRI of the brain, because this technique allows good visualization of the posterior fossa. If these changes are visualized, then the condition is most likely chronic (as also indicated by the history), and most likely irreversible. However, it is important to make sure that the patient is well nourished, takes vitamins, and stops drinking in order to prevent other neurologic problems from occurring. Damage to other brain regions listed do not cause such damage.

**465. The answer is b.** *(Kandel, 3/e, pp 632–642.)* The spinocerebellum receives sensory inputs from the spinal cord and is instrumental in controlling posture and movement. It includes the vermis and the intermediate hemisphere. The cerebrocerebellum consists of the lateral hemispheres and is instrumental in the planning of movement. The dentate nucleus comprises the cell bodies that form the brachium conjunctivum. The brachium conjunctivum and pontis correspond to the superior and middle cerebellar peduncles, respectively.

**466. The answer is e.** *(Kandel, 3/e, pp 635–637.)* The spinocerebellar cortical (Purkinje) cells project to the fastigial and interposed nuclei.

**467. The answer is e.** *(Kandel, 3/e, p 635.)* Purkinje cells are found in the cerebellar cortex. None of the other choices are cells found in the cerebellum.

**468. The answer is b.** (*Rowland, 9/e, pp 294–302.*) This case is an example of a condition called "normal pressure hydrocephalus." This may be caused by various nonprogressive meningeal and ependymal diseases such as chronic meningitis and subarachnoid hemorrhages, which can initially block CSF absorption. Initially the CSF pressure is high, which results in the enlargement of the ventricles. The CSF pressure becomes normal because the CSF absorption begins again. However, the enlarged ventricles, despite normal CSF pressure, cause hydrostatic impairment to the central white matter surrounding the ventricles. Maximal ventricular expansion is usually located in the frontal lobes with preservation of the cortical gray matter and other subcortical structures. As a result, patients with this condition have diminished frontal lobe functions, namely gait problems without any weakness, as well as urinary incontinence and dementia. Frontal lobe dysfunction can also cause the reappearance of primitive reflexes that disappear shortly after birth, such as the grasp reflex. Late in the course of normal pressure hydrocephalus, the patient may develop "frontal lobe incontinence," where he or she becomes indifferent to the incontinence, much like a very small child. Headaches are rare in this particular type of hydrocephalus. Normal pressure hydrocephalus is usually diagnosed with a thorough neurological examination, in addition to a head CT (computerized tomography), which shows enlarged ventricles and occasionally interstitial fluid within the white matter adjacent to the lateral ventricles. Measurement of CSF pressures with a lumbar puncture, and radionuclide cisternography (a procedure where a radionuclide is injected intrathecally, and its distribution is observed over a period of 24 hours) are also helpful. Occasionally, shunting procedures that allow the CSF to drain into the peritoneal cavity or the blood are helpful if performed early in the course of this condition.

**469. The answer is c.** (*Rowland, 9/e, pp 294–302.*) The major mechanism underlying hydrocephalus is decreased absorption of CSF. In the case of normal pressure hydrocephalus, the problem is described above (see answer for the previous question). Another cause of decreased absorption is obstruction of CSF flow by a tumor. Low blood pressure does not cause enlarged ventricles. High blood pressure only causes hydrocephalus as a result of hypertensive crisis, but not chronically. Decreased blood flow in the brain can actually be used as a temporizing measure to acutely decrease intracranial pressure in emergencies, in order to make room for expanding tissue through the mechanism of decreasing $pCO_2$ in the brain with a ventilator.

**470. The answer is c.** (*Rowland, 9/e, pp 294–302.*) The major location for reabsorption of CSF is the arachnoid villi within the ventricular system. In the case of this particular patient, there is a history of a subarachnoid hemorrhage, which may have caused obstruction within this area.

**471. The answer is e.** (*Rowland, 9/e, pp 294–302.*) The frontal horns of the lateral ventricles are the area of greatest expansion; thus the expansion would affect the adjoining white matter of the frontal lobe. The other areas listed are subcortical and gray matter areas, which are located further from the expanding frontal horns, and less affected. The pituitary gland is quite distant from the frontal horns as well.

**472. The answer is c.** (*Rowland, 9/e, pp 8–10, 56–58.*) The language problem is an example of Broca's aphasia, a deficit seen with lesions of Broca's area and manifested by defects in the "motor" aspect of speech, leaving the patient's speech halting and nonfluent. People with Broca's aphasia tend to repeat certain phrases, as well as leave out pronouns. Since the language centers are usually located on the dominant side of the brain (the left side for a right-handed person), this lesion must be on the left side of Joe's brain. Wernicke's aphasia is a problem with the sensory aspect of speech, where the patient can speak fluently, but the speech sounds like gibberish. The area of disruption in this type of aphasia is usually in Wernicke's area, a region of the posterior superior temporal lobe. Dysarthria is slurred speech, but makes grammatical sense. Alexia is the inability to read. Pure word deafness is a type of sensory aphasia where language, reading, and writing are only mildly disturbed, but auditory comprehension of words is very abnormal. This arises from lesions of the posterior temporal lobe.

**473. The answer is e.** (*Rowland, 9/e, pp 8–10, 56–58.*) Joe's condition is an example of a left inferior frontal lobe cortical stroke including the region of Broca's area and the left precentral gyrus. The weakness on his right side confirms this, since the left side of the brain controls the right side of the body. The right leg is most likely less involved than the arm because the "leg" area of the precentral gyrus extends onto the medial aspect of the frontal lobe, an area served by a different artery than that serving the "arm" and "face" areas. The internal capsule contains motor fibers traveling to the cortex, but usually does not involve language. The thalamus contains many sensory, motor, and association areas, but only rarely causes language problems. Functions of the pontine reticular formation do not include language. The corpus callosum is a white matter structure which connects the hemispheres. Lesions of the posterior aspect may cause language problems, such as alexia without agraphia (the ability to write, but not to read), but would not cause both an aphasia as well as weakness.

**474. The answer is d.** *(Rowland, 9/e, pp 8–10, 56–58.)* The middle cerebral artery subserves the precentral gyrus, the area which has been damaged. The damage can be more widespread, depending upon which portion of the vessel becomes occluded. The anterior cerebral artery supplies the orbitofrontal cortex, deep limbic structures, as well as the cingulate gyrus. The posterior cerebral artery supplies the thalamus, portions of the temporal lobes, and portions of the midbrain. The anterior inferior cerebellar artery supplies the lateral inferior pons and portions of the cerebellum. Perforating branches of the basilar artery supply medial portions of the brainstem. The irregular heart beat observed in this case is an example of aerial fibrillation, a heart rhythm which is often recognized by being "irregularly irregular." This rhythm can cause strokes by throwing small blood clots or emboli from the heart to the cerebral blood vessels and occluding them.

**475. The answer is b.** *(Rowland, 9/e, pp 8–10, 56–58.)* Joe's forehead doesn't droop like the rest of his face because this region receives innervation from both sides of the cerebral cortex, giving this area a "back-up" in case of damage. This can only occur when the lesion is above the level of the VII nerve, where both sides no longer contribute to the innervation of the face. This type of weakness is called a central VII nerve lesion, because it occurs within the central nervous system. A peripheral VII nerve lesion is a lesion within the VII nerve nucleus, or distal. This type of lesion always involves the forehead in addition to the rest of the face. The XII nerve innervates the tongue, the V nerve innervates sensation of the face, in addition to the muscles of mastication, but not the muscles of facial expression. The oculomotor nerve innervates 4 of the muscles which move the eyes.

**476. The answer is a.** *(Rowland, 9/e, pp 8–10, 56–58.)* Joe is probably right-handed, which implies left-sided cerebral dominance. Since language is usually on the dominant side, and Joe has an aphasia, his dominant cerebral hemisphere has been damaged. People who are left-handed may also have dominance of either side, or may have mixed dominance. True ambidexterity is rare.

**477. The answer is a.** (*Adams, 6/e, pp 676–678.*) The MRI of Susan's head revealed a pituitary microadenoma, a benign tumor arising from the anterior pituitary or adenohypophysis. This particular tumor consisted of cells that secrete the hormone prolactin, which is not only the stimulating factor for lactation but inhibits menstruation when levels are high. It is common for this tumor's symptoms to be manifested during the child-bearing years.

**478. The answer is c.** (*Kandel, 3/e, p 437. Adams, 6/e, pp 247–251.*) The visual problem is called bitemporal hemianopsia. Since the pituitary gland is in very close proximity to the optic chiasm, pituitary tumors often invade this structure. Since only the medial fibers (which perceive the temporal field of each eye) in each optic nerve cross, these are the fibers damaged by these tumors, and the patient will be unable to see either temporal visual field. Both central scotoma (an island of visual loss surrounded by normal vision in one eye), which is usually seen with lesions of the retina or optic nerve, and papilledema (blurring of the optic disc margin when viewed by funduscopic examination due to increased intracranial pressure) would not be caused by damage to the optic chiasm.

**479. The answer is d.** (*Kandel, 3/e, p 437.*) The optic chiasm can be compressed by pituitary tumors, causing bitemporal hemianopsia (see answer for previous question).

**480. The answer is e.** (*Kandel, 3/e, p 863.*) Prolactin-releasing factor is found in the arcuate nucleus of the hypothalamus, and activates the lactotrophic cells of the anterior pituitary gland.

**481. The answer is a.** (*Kandel, 3/e, p 863.*) Several different peptides, including dopamine, have the capacity to raise the level of prolactin in the blood. Specifically, the tuberoinfundibular dopaminergic system regulates prolactin secretion through direct projection to the pituitary. For this reason, a newer treatment for prolactin-secreting microadenomas is the drug bromocriptine, a dopamine agonist commonly used in the treatment of

Parkinson's disease. By giving a dopamine agonist, serum prolactin increases, inhibiting production by the tumor cells, and eventually the tumor shrinks. This has become either an alternative, or first-line treatment, prior to trying radiation or surgery.

**482. The answer is b.** (*Wilson-Pauwels, pp 26–33.*) The third cranial nerve (oculomotor) controls four of the six extraocular muscles that move the eye. When this nerve fails to function, the eye remains deviated laterally due to the unopposed action of the other two extraocular muscles. When the eyes no longer move together, patients have double vision because the visual cortex now receives two different images. In addition, fibers originating in the third nerve nucleus innervate the levator palpebrae superioris, a muscle which helps to lift the eyelid. Damage to the optic nerve causes loss of vision, blurred vision, and a central scotoma (blind spot in the center of the visual field). Damage to the cervical sympathetic fibers causes *Horner's syndrome*, consisting of ptosis (drooping of the eyelid), miosis (constriction of the pupil), and anhydrosis (loss of sweating), not eye movement abnormalities. The actions of the superior oblique, (the muscle innervated by the trochlear nerve) include intorsion, depression, and abduction. The abducens nerve mediates the lateral rectus muscle, which abducts the eye.

**483. The answer is c.** (*Wilson-Pauwels, pp 26–33.*) The eye is depressed and abducted due the unopposed actions of the superior oblique and lateral rectus muscles, which together move the eye downward, and abduct it (see above for the actions of these muscles). The other four muscles are innervated by the oculomotor nerve, which presumably has been damaged.

**484. The answer is e.** (*Kandel, 3/e, p 728. Adams, 6/e, p 795.*) This is an example of Weber syndrome, or a lesion involving the third cranial nerve outflow tract, and the corticospinal and corticobulbar tracts in the cerebral peduncles of the midbrain. Weber syndrome may occur as a result of an occlusion of the interpeduncular branches of the posterior cerebral artery which supply this portion of the midbrain, a tumor pressing on this area, an aneurysm (circumscribed dilation of an artery) of the posterior communicating artery, or a plaque (lesion) related to multiple sclerosis.

**485. The answer is c.** (*Wilson-Pauwels, pp 34–36.*) Fibers from the Edinger-Westphal nucleus are affected by a lesion of the midbrain, as well, and because they are instrumental in constricting the pupil, this lesion causes the patient to have a dilated pupil. If there is a mass external to the midbrain, but pressing on the oculomotor nerve, then the preganglionic parasympathetic fibers traveling to the ciliary ganglion—which in turn, innervate the pupillary constrictor muscles—can be damaged, also causing a dilated pupil. Cervical sympathetic fibers cause pupillary dilatation, so damage to these fibers causes pupillary constriction (see Horner's syndrome, above).

**486. The answer is e.** *(Kandel, 3/e, p 728. Adams, 6/e, p 795.)* Involvement of the cerebral peduncle causes damage to the corticospinal and corticobulbar tracts, resulting in weakness of the contralateral face, arm, and leg. The motor deficit is contralateral because the corticospinal tracts cross in the medullary pyramids, below the level of the lesion. The upper portion of Mike's face was spared in this case (as well as in any other upper motor neuron lesion) because the face is innervated bilaterally until the level of the caudal pons, so a unilateral lesion results in sparing of this portion of the face. The combination of a third nerve palsy and contralateral hemiparesis can only occur in the midbrain. The observed effects relating to cranial nerve III could not be accounted for by cortical damage. Likewise, damage to the cervical cord would not effect the third nerve, as well.

**487. The answer is d.** *(Adams, 6/e, p 347.)* The CT scan of Louise's brain revealed a large, acute stroke of her upper pons and midbrain. Strokes of these areas often result from occlusion of the basilar artery and can produce coma, or a variant of hypersomnia called akinetic mutism or coma vigil. An EEG of a patient like this shows a pattern associated with slow wave sleep, but eye movements are preserved.

**488. The answer is a.** *(Kandel, 3/e, p 1047.)* It is likely that the corticospinal tracts within the pons were damaged during this very large stroke, causing the increased tone from lack of inhibition, as well as the lack of movement in Louise's arms and legs.

**489. The answer is d.** *(Kandel, 3/e, pp 726–728, 815–816.)* Infarctions of perforators of the basilar artery, supplying the reticular formation of the pons, may cause coma. These perforators also supply the corticospinal tracts, causing the increased tone and weakness of Louise's legs, so a large stroke may involve both functions.

**490. The answer is c.** (*Adams, 6/e, p 350.*) Coma occurs because there is damage to the brainstem tegmentum, which is a major component of the ascending reticular activating system. Although it is not known exactly which area is precisely responsible for consciousness, lesions of this region, as well as projections from the medial regions of the midbrain reticular formation, can produce coma.

**491. The answer is e.** (*Kandel, 3/e, pp 693–698.*) The two main monoaminergic systems of the reticular formation are the noradrenergic and serotonergic systems, originating in the locus ceruleus and raphe nuclei, respectively. The mesolimbic, mesostriatal, and mesocortical dopaminergic systems are located within the ventro-rostral aspect of the brainstem, but not within the reticular formation. Melatonin is found in the pineal gland, not in the reticular formation.

**492. The answer is d.** (*Kandel, 3/e, p 388.*) Norma's head CT showed an old stroke in her left ventral thalamus, and no new lesions. A stroke involving the ventral posterolateral nucleus of the thalamus, especially several months after the stroke, can produce an entity called the syndrome of Dejerine-Roussy, or "thalamic pain syndrome." Although there is sensory loss on the contralateral side, there is pain or discomfort out of proportion to the stimulus on the affected side of the body. Emotional disturbance aggravates the response. Some patients describe the sensation as "knife-like" or "hot." As the deficit (numbness) resolves, the pain may lessen. This syndrome may also occur in lesions of the parietal white matter, and is thought to occur as a result of an imbalance of afferent sensory impulses.

**493. The answer is b.** (*Kandel, 3/e, pp 363, 707.*) Sensation of the limbs and trunk are projected through the ventral posterior lateral nucleus of the thalamus to the somatosensory cortex. Sensory information from the face is carried through the trigeminal system to the ventral posterior medial nucleus, from which it is projected to the somatosensory cortex.

**494. The answer is d.** (*Kandel, 3/e, p 362.*) The spinothalamic tract is the only sensory pathway listed that mediates pain.

**495. The answer is e.** (*Kandel, 3/e, p 393.*) The periaqueductal gray is one area of many which produces analgesia when stimulated in both animals and in humans. It is an area with a high density of opiate receptors and opioidergic neurons, and is thought to represent a key area in gating pain.

**496. The answer is e.** (*Kandel, 3/e, pp 394–396.*) Many neurotransmitters have been implicated as pain modulators, including the opiates and enkephalins, norepinephrine, serotonin, substance P, GABA, and acetylcholine. Most analgesic medications are designed to target a particular aspect of the pain pathway. In more recent years, the advent of a class of drugs called tricyclic antidepressants has added another dimension to medical pain treatment. The methylated forms of these medications are useful blockers of serotonin reuptake. Since serotonin is known to be a pain modulator, it is thought that blocking the reuptake of serotonin enhances its action and facilitates the action of intrinsic opiates to relieve pain. This is a common class of drugs used to treat chronic pain, since these medications are not addictive.

**497. The answer is c.** (*Wilson-Pauwels, p 47.*) Damage to the trochlear nerve causes weakness of the superior oblique muscle, resulting in the inability of the orbit to deviate downward when the eye is intorted. In order to compensate for the classically vertical double vision, the patient tends to tilt his head to the contralateral side, causing the contralateral eye to intort.

**498. The answer is d.** (*Wilson-Pauwels, pp 45–47.*) The trochlear nerve supplies the superior oblique muscle.

**499. The answer is b.** (*Wilson-Pauwels, pp 43–44.*) The trochlear nerve is the only nerve to decussate peripherally, and also, to emerge from the dorsal aspect of the brainstem. In this case, the damaged nerve emerged from the right (contralateral) dorsal midbrain.

**500. The answer is d.** (*Wilson-Pauwels, p 46.*) The action of the superior oblique muscle is to rotate the eye medially and downward.

**501. The answer is e.** (*Adams, 6/e, p 270.*) Because the trochlear is not only the smallest cranial nerve, but also has the longest course of any cranial nerve, it is especially vulnerable to trauma. One of the most common causes of trochlear nerve palsy is trauma.

# HIGH-YIELD FACTS

# HIGH-YIELD FACTS

## Gross Anatomy of the Brain

1. Lateral view of the brain. The loci of key motor and sensory structures of the cerebral cortex are indicated in the figure shown below. Anatomical definitions: anterior—toward the front (rostral end) of the forebrain; posterior—toward the back (caudal end) of the forebrain; dorsal—toward the superior surface of the forebrain; ventral—toward the inferior surface of the forebrain. Note that with respect to the brainstem and spinal cord, the terms *anterior* and *ventral* are synonymous, and likewise, *posterior* and *dorsal* are also synonymous. Here, the term *rostral* means toward the midbrain, and the term *caudal* means toward the sacral aspect of spinal cord.

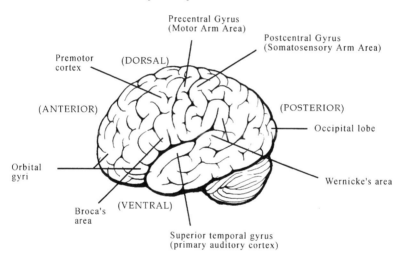

2. Midsagittal view of the brain shown on p. 228. Magnetic resonance image: T2-weighted, high resolution, fast spin echo image (Courtesy of Leo J. Wolansky, M.D.).

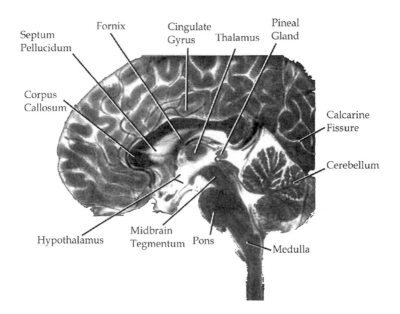

Septum Pellucidum — Fornix — Cingulate Gyrus — Thalamus — Pineal Gland

Corpus Callosum

Calcarine Fissure

Cerebellum

Hypothalamus — Midbrain Tegmentum — Pons — Medulla

3. Horizontal (transaxial) view of the brain shown opposite. Magnetic resonance image: Fast inversion recovery for myelin suppression image (Courtesy of Leo J. Wolansky, M.D.).

4. Frontal view of the brain shown on p. 230. Magnetic resonance image: Fast inversion recovery for myelin suppression image (Courtesy of Leo J. Wolansky, M.D.).

## Table I
### Structures Identified in Figures 1-4 and Their Functions

| Structure | Function |
| --- | --- |
| Precentral gyrus | Primary motor cortex—mediates voluntary movements associated with individual muscle groups |
| Premotor cortex | Component of the corticospinal system—integrates complex movements of the eyes, body, and head and is dependent upon sensory inputs |
| Orbital gyri | Part of the prefrontal cortex—mediates higher intellectual functions and emotional behavior |
| Broca's area | Left side of inferior frontal cortex—important for expression of speech |

| Superior temporal gyrus | Primary auditory receiving area |
|---|---|
| Wernicke's area | Left side of temporal and adjoining parietal cortices—important for comprehension of speech |
| Occipital lobe | Visual receiving area—key regions including areas 17, 18, and 19 |
| Postcentral gyrus | Primary somatosensory receiving area |
| Fornix | Primary output pathway of the hippocampal formation to the septal area and diencephalon |
| Septum pellucidum | A thin plate separating the lateral ventricles on each side of brain; in lower forms, this region (called the septal area) contains many cells and fibers that project to the hypothalamus and mediates visceral, autonomic, and emotional functions associated with the hypothalamus |

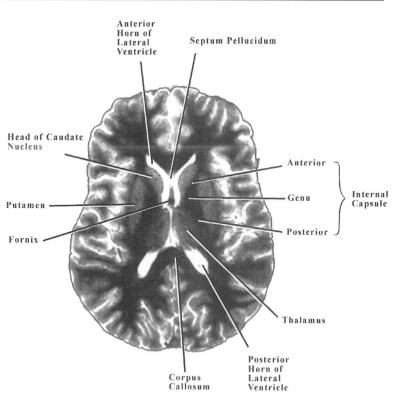

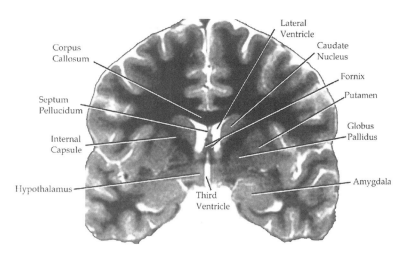

## Table I (Cont.)

| Structure | Function |
| --- | --- |
| Corpus callosum | Commissural pathway connecting different regions of both sides of the cortex |
| Hypothalamus | Situated in ventral aspect of diencephalon—mediates visceral functions such as autonomic, endocrine, temperature regulation, feeding, drinking, aggression, and rage |
| Midbrain tegmentum | Dorsal aspect of pons and middle region of midbrain—mediates autonomic, sensory and motor functions |
| Pons | Consists of a basilar portion and tegmentum—mediates autonomic, sensory, and motor functions, including those associated with cranial nerves |
| Medulla | Most caudal part of brainstem adjoining the spinal cord—contains major ascending and descending tracts and mediates autonomic, sensory and motor functions, including those associated with cranial nerves |
| Cerebellum | Key structure for the coordination of motor responses |
| Calcarine fissure | Part of the occipital cortex; on the lower and upper banks of this fissure lie the receiving areas for visual inputs associated with upper and lower visual fields, respectively |

| | |
|---|---|
| Pineal gland | An endocrine gland linked to the regulation of circadian rhythms; it secretes serotonin, melatonin, norepinephrine, somatostatin, and hypothalamic-releasing hormones |
| Thalamus | Situated in dorsal two thirds of diencephalon; a primary source of inputs to the cerebral cortex |
| Cingulate gyrus | A component of the limbic system; provides inputs to the hippocampal formation and has been implicated in such functions as autonomic regulation, rage, aggression and memory |
| Caudate nucleus | A major receiving area of the basal ganglia whose principal inputs are from cerebral cortex |
| Putamen | A second major receiving area of the basal ganglia whose principal inputs are from cerebral cortex and centre median nucleus of the thalamus |
| Lateral ventricle | Located in the forebrain; contains a posterior horn, body, inferior horn, and anterior horn; much of the CSF produced in the brain is derived from the choroid plexus of the lateral ventricle |
| Internal capsule | Transmits mainly descending fibers from the cerebral cortex to the brainstem and spinal cord; contains an anterior horn, genu, and posterior horn; fibers contained within the anterior horn arise from frontal lobe and project to pons; fibers situated in the genu arise from the ventral aspect of precentral gyrus (head region) and project to brainstem; fibers associated with posterior horn arise from the hemisphere of the precentral gyrus (arm and leg region) and project to spinal cord |
| Third ventricle | Located in diencephalon; receives CSF from lateral ventricle and transports CSF to the fourth ventricle via the cerebral aqueduct |
| Globus pallidus | Contains the major output neurons of the basal ganglia, which project to the cerebral cortex via ventrolateral, ventral anterior, centre median nuclei of thalamus |

## DEVELOPMENT

5.  The primitive nervous system is divided into two regions by the sulcus limitans: an alar plate, from which sensory regions of the spinal cord and brain

stem are formed, and a basal plate, from which motor regions of the spinal cord and brainstem are formed.

## THE NEURON

6. Activation of sodium channels is associated with membrane depolarization, while activation of potassium and chloride channels is associated with membrane hyperpolarization. After information is received from a presynaptic neuron, depolarization occurs in the postsynaptic neuron; then the action potential is initiated and propagated down the axon from the initial segment.

7. Myelin formation is produced in the peripheral nervous system by numerous Schwann cells, while a similar function in the central nervous system is carried out by an oligodendrocyte, which can wrap itself around numbers of neurons. Myelination in the nervous system allows for rapid conduction of action potentials by a process of saltatory conduction, in which the signals skip along openings in the myelin called nodes of Ranvier. Damage to the such myelinated neurons typically disrupts the transmission of neural signals and is frequently seen in autoimmune diseases such as multiple sclerosis, in which sensory and motor functions are severely compromised.

## THE SYNAPSE and NEUROTRANSMITTERS

8. The sequence of events in synaptic transmission is: transmitter synthesis → presynaptic potential → release of transmitter into synaptic cleft → binding of transmitter to postsynaptic receptor → postsynaptic potential → removal of transmitter.

9. Major excitatory transmitters: Substance P, acetylcholine, and excitatory amino acids; major inhibitory transmitters: GABA, enkephalin, and glycine. Disruption of neurotransmitter function can lead to different diseases of the nervous system. One such example involves the role of acetylcholine at the neuromuscular junction. When antibodies are formed against the acetylcholine receptor at the neuromuscular junction, transmission is disrupted and the autoimmune disease called myasthenia gravis occurs. This disorder includes symptoms such as weakness and fatigue of the muscles.

## SPINAL CORD

10.                          **Table II**
              **Major Ascending Tracts of the Spinal Cord**

| Major Ascending Tracts | Functions |
| --- | --- |
| Dorsal columns | mediates conscious proprioception, 2-pt. discrimination, some tactile sensation: dorsal columns → ipsilateral dorsal column nuclei → contralateral VPL nucleus of thalamus → postcentral gyrus |
| Lateral spinothalamic tract | mediates pain and temperature: spinothalamic tract neurons → contralateral VPL and posterior complex of thalamus → postcentral gyrus |
| Anterior spinothalamic tract | mediates tactile impulses: anterior spinothalamic tract neurons → contralateral VPL → postcentral gyrus |
| Posterior spinocerebellar tract | mediates unconscious proprioception from muscle spindles and Golgi tendon organs of lower limbs: posterior spinocerebellar tract (from n. Dorsalis) via inferior cerebellar peduncle → ipsilateral anterior lobe of cerebellum |
| Cuneocerebellar tract | mediates unconscious proprioception from muscle spindles and Golgi tendon organs of upper limbs: ascending fibers in dorsal columns → accessory cuneate nucleus → (via inferior cerebellar peduncle) to ipsilateral anterior lobe of cerebellum |
| Anterior spinocerebellar tract | mediates unconscious proprioception from Golgi tendon organ of lower limbs: spinal cord neurons decussate → to anterior lobe of cerebellum (bilaterally) via superior cerebellar peduncle |

11.

**Table III**
**Major Descending Tracts of the Spinal Cord**

| Major Descending Tracts | Functions |
|---|---|
| Lateral corticospinal tract | mediates voluntary control of motor functions: primary motor, premotor, supplementary motor and postcentral gyrus via internal capsule, crus cerebri and pyramids crossed → all levels of spinal cord |
| Rubrospinal tract | mediates excitation of flexor motor neurons: red nucleus via ventral tegmental decussation → contralateral spinal cord at cervical and lumbar levels |
| Lateral reticulospinal tract | mediates inhibition of spinal reflexes (mainly of extensors): medial medullary neurons descend bilaterally → cervical and lumbar levels of spinal cord |
| Medial reticulospinal tract | mediates excitation of spinal reflexes (mainly of extensors): medial pontine neurons descend ipsilaterally → cervical and lumbar levels of spinal cord |
| Lateral vestibulospinal tract | mediates excitation of extensor motor neurons: lateral vestibular neurons descend ipsilaterally → cervical and lumbar levels of spinal cord |
| Medial vestibulospinal tract | mediates regulation of postural reflexes of head and neck: medial vestibular neurons descend via MLF → cervical levels of spinal cord |

12.

**Table IV**
**Major Disorders of the Spinal Cord**

| Disease | Affected Structure(s) | Description of Loss |
|---|---|---|
| Brown-Sequard syndrome | Hemisection of spinal cord (dueoften to a knife or bullet wound) | Contralateral loss of pain and temperature below level of lesion; bilateral segmental loss of pain and temperature at level of lesion; ipsilateral loss of conscious proprioception; ipsilateral upper motor neuron paralysis below level of lesion; ipsilateral lower motor neuron paralysis at level of lesion |
| Tabes Dorsalis | Damage to dorsal root ganglia and dorsal (often resulting from syphilis) | Ipsilateral loss of conscious proprioception and tendon reflexes |
| Amyotrophic Lateral Sclerosis (ALS) | Etiology is unknown; loss of corticospinal fibers and ventral horn cells | Abnormal reflexes, muscle weakness, atrophy of muscles, and ultimate death |
| Syringomyelia | Damage to spinothalamic fibers caused by abnormal closure of central canal during development, by trauma, or by tumor. If the syrinx becomes larger, the ventral horn gray matter may become involved | Segmental loss of pain and temperature. Expansion of the syrinx to the ventral horn gray matter would cause a lower motor neuron paralysis |
| Combined Systems Disease | Degeneration of both dorsal columns and corticospinal tracts due to pernicious anemia associated with deficiency in vitamin B12 | Loss of conscious proprioception, position sense, upper motor neuron symptoms, and muscle weakness |

## AUTONOMIC NERVOUS SYSTEM

13. The sympathetic nervous system arises from the thoracic and lumbar cords ($T_1$ - $L_2$) and the parasympathetic nervous system arises from $S_2$ - $S_4$ and cranial nerves III, VII, IX, and X. All preganglionic neurons are cholinergic as well as parasympathetic postganglionic neurons. In addition, sympathetic postganglionic innervation of sweat glands and blood vessels in skeletal muscle is also cholinergic. Most other postganglionic sympathetic endings are adrenergic. Examples of functions of the sympathetic nervous system include: pupillary dilation, acceleration of heart rate, constriction of blood vessels of the trunk and extremities, and inhibition of gastric motility. Examples of functions of the parasympathetic nervous system include: pupillary constriction, decrease in heart rate, secretion of salivary and lacrimal glands, and stimulation of gastric motility.

## THE BRAINSTEM AND CRANIAL NERVES

14. **Lateral medullary (Wallenberg's syndrome):** occlusion of the inferior cerebellar arteries cause lesions of the lateral aspect of the lower half of the brainstem, producing loss of pain and temperature on the same side of the face and opposite side of the body, as well as Horner's syndrome (i.e., miosis, ptosis, and decreased sweating on one side of face due to disruption of the sympathetic supply to the orbit and pupil, or, as applies in the present context, to disruption of descending sympathetic fibers through the brainstem to the spinal cord).

15. **Medial medullary syndrome:** occlusion of the anterior spinal artery causes lesions of the medial aspect of the medulla, producing contralateral loss of conscious proprioception, contralateral hemiparesis, and weakness of tongue muscles that are protruded to side of lesion. Body paralysis, which involves the side contralateral to the lesion, coupled with cranial nerve weakness, which involves the side ipsilateral to lesion, is called "alternating hypoglossal hemiplegia."

16. Cranial nerves mediate multiple functions in the nervous system. Motor nuclei: general somatic efferent (NIII, NIV, NVI, NXII), special visceral efferent (NV, NVII, NIX, NX, NXI), general visceral efferent (NIII, NVII, NIX, NX), general somatic afferent (NV, NIX, NX), special sensory afferent (NII, NVIII), or special visceral afferent (NI, NVII, NIX, NX).

17.

**Table V**
**Summary of Anatomical and Functional Properties of Cranial Nerves**

| Cranial Nerve | Type | Peripheral Component | Central | Major Projections | Dysfunctions |
|---|---|---|---|---|---|
| I. Olfactory | SVA | olfactory mucosa | olfactory bulb | olfactory bulb projections to temporal lobe and limbic system | loss of sense of smell; olfactory hallucinations from temporal lobe lesions |
| II. Optic nerve | SSA | retina | lateral geniculate nucleus; pretectal region; superior colliculus | lateral geniculate fibers to the occipital cortex; vision and visual reflexes | varying degrees of blindness depending upon the extent of retinal or optic nerve damage; loss of pupillary light reflex |
| III. Oculomotor nerve | GSE | | oculomotor nucleus (midbrain) | innervates extraocular eye muscles (except lateral rectus and superior oblique); levator palpebrae superior | medial gaze paralysis, loss of convergence, loss of up and down movement |
| | GVE | | Edinger-Westphal Nucleus (midbrain) | preganglionic parasymp. neurons → ciliary gang → pupillary sphincter (constriction of pupil) and ciliary muscles (bulging of lens) | loss of pupillary light reflex; dilated pupil |

## Table V (Cont.)

| Cranial Nerve | Type | Component Peripheral | Component Central | Major Projections | Dysfunctions |
|---|---|---|---|---|---|
| IV. Trochlear nerve | GSE | | trochlear nucleus (midbrain) | innervates superior oblique muscle; bring eye down when in medial position | double vision when looking downward; eye cannot be pulled downward when in medial position |
| V. Trigeminal nerve | GSA | semilunar ganglion | main sensory and spinal nucleus; mesencephalic nucleus (upper pons) | 1st order neurons transmit pain/ temperature fibers from head and ant. two thirds of tongue to spinal nucleus; pressure, touch, conscious proprioception to main sensory nucleus; projections then go to VPM of thalamus; muscle spindles to mesencephalic nucleus | loss of somatic sensation from the region of the head |
| | SVE | | motor nucleus (pons) | innervates masticatory muscles for jaw closing responses | difficulty in chewing; loss of jaw closing responses |

| Nerve | Component | Ganglion | Nucleus | Function | Deficit |
|---|---|---|---|---|---|
| VI. Abducens nerve | GSE | | abducens nucleus (pons) | innervates lateral rectus muscle (lateral movement of eye) | lateral gaze paralysis; double vision on attempts at lateral gaze |
| VII. Facial nerve | SVE | | facial nucleus (pons) | innervates muscles of facial expression | loss of facial expression; loss of corneal reflex |
| | GVE | | superior salivatory nucleus | preganglionic parasymp. neurons → submandib., pterygopalatine ganglion → submandibular; sublingual, lacrimal, nasal, and palatine glands | loss of salivary responses; loss of lacrimation |
| | SVA | geniculate ganglion | solitary nucleus | taste inputs from anterior two-thirds of tongue to solitary nucleus → VPM | loss of taste sensation from anterior two thirds of the tongue |
| | GSA | geniculate ganglion | spinal nucleus of N. V | cutaneous sensation from pinna of ear → spinal nucleus → VPM | loss of sensation from small region around pinna and back of ear |
| VIII. Auditory-vestibular nerve | SSA | spiral ganglion (audit.) | auditory nuclei in upper medulla | auditory projections from basilar membrane through relay nuclei in pons, midbrain and thalamus to the superior temporal gyrus | loss of hearing |

**Table V (Cont.)**

| Cranial Nerve | Type | Component Peripheral | Component Central | Major Projections | Dysfunctions |
|---|---|---|---|---|---|
| | SSA | Scarpa's Ganglion (vestib.) | vestibular nuclei | vestibular inputs from semicircular canals and otolith organ to vestibular nuclei; inputs to N. III, IV, and VI for regulation of eye movements and to cerebellum for maintenance of balance | loss of balance; loss of vestibulo-ocular reflex; loss of labyrinthine reflexes; nystagmus; dizziness; nausea |
| IX. *Glossopharyngeal nerve* | SVE | | nucleus ambiguus | innervates stylopharyngeus muscle (pharynx) | impairment of gag, uvular, and palatal reflexes |
| | GVE | | inferior salivatory nucleus | preganglionic parasymp. → otic ganglion → parotid gland (salivation) | loss of salivation |
| | SVA | inferior ganglion | solitary nucleus; | taste from posterior third of tongue | loss of taste from posterior tongue |

| | | | | |
|---|---|---|---|---|
| | inferior ganglion | reticular formation | signals oxygen tension in blood; chemoreceptor inputs from carotid body to retic. format → increases in respiration | disruption of respiratory reflexes |
| GVA | inferior ganglion | solitary nucleus | increases in blood pressure from carotid sinus → solitary n. → dorsal motor n. → slowing of heart | loss of homeostatic reflex mechanism for control of blood pressure |
| GSA | superior ganglion | spinal nucleus (N.V) | cutaneous sensation from skin of external ear and posterior third of tongue | loss of general sensation from posterior third of tongue |
| X. *Vagus nerve* SVE | | nucleus ambiguus | motor innervation of the pharynx, larynx and soft palate; important for phonation and swallowing | loss of swallowing; hoarseness and aphonia; lesion can be fatal because of asphyxia due to constriction of laryngeal muscles |

**Table V (Cont.)**

| Cranial Nerve | Type | Component Peripheral | Central | Major Projections | Dysfunctions |
|---|---|---|---|---|---|
| | GVE | | dorsal motor nucleus | innervation of the heart and other body viscera → produces slowing of heart, speed of peristalsis, and increase in visceral secretions | hyperactivity produces ulcers; loss of carotid sinus reflex |
| | SVA | inferior ganglion | solitary nucleus | taste impulses from the epiglottis | ? |
| | SVA | inferior ganglion | reticular formation | chemoreceptors in aortic body signal oxygen changes in blood → reticular formation → descending pathway to thoracic cord for increases in respiration | disruption of respiratory reflexes |
| | GVA | inferior ganglion | solitary nucleus | stretch receptors in aortic arch signal increases in blood pressure to solitary nucleus → dorsal motor n. → vagal slowing of heart | loss of homeostatic reflex for control of blood pressure |

| | | | | |
|---|---|---|---|---|
| | GSA | superior ganglion | spinal nucleus (N.V) | cutaneous sensation from back of ear ext. auditory canal → spinal n. (N.V) → VPM | possible loss of general sensation from region innervated |
| XI. *Spinal accessory nerve* | SVE | | C1-C6 of spinal cord | nerves innervate sternomastoid and trapezius → contralateral turning and lifting of head | difficulty in raising head and moving it to opposite side; sagging of shoulder |
| XII. *Hypoglossal nerve* | GSE | | hypoglossal nucleus | innervates muscles of the tongue; controls shape and position of tongue | lower motor neuron paralysis produces deviation of tongue to ipsilateral side of lesion; upper motor neuron lesion produces deviation of tongue to contralateral side of lesion |

18.

## Table VI
### Summary of Cranial Nerve Reflexes

| Cranial Nerve(s) | Name of Reflex | Description |
|---|---|---|
| Nerves II & III | pupillary light reflex | constriction of pupil in presence of light: optic nerve and tract → pretectal area → N. III → preganglionic parasymp. → ciliary ganglion → postganglionic fibers to pupillary constrictor muscles |
| Nerves II & III | accommodation | medial convergence, pupillary constriction and focussing onto a near object: optic nerve and tract to lateral geniculate nucleus → visual cortex → pretectal area → N. III (GSE and GVE components) → medial rectus muscle & Edinger-Westphal nucleus → ciliary ganglion → ciliary muscle → bulging of lens and pupillary constrictor muscles → constriction of pupil |
| Nerves III & VIII | vestibulo-ocular reflex | smooth pursuit and saccadic eye movements (nystagmus): vestibular inputs due to sudden turning of head → vestibular nuclei via MLF → pontine gaze center → contralateral N.III and ipsilateral N. VI → medial rectus (contralateral) and lateral rectus (ipsilateral) → horizontal movements of the eyes |
| Nerves V & VII | corneal reflex | irritation of the cornea causes closing of the eye: ophthalmic branch of N.V → motor nucleus of N. VII → orbicularis oris m. → closing of eye |
| Nerve V | jaw jerk (masseter reflex) | tapping of the chin of slightly opened mouth results in a jaw closing response: muscle spindle activation of lower jaw muscles → afferent fiber of N. V to mesencephalic nucleus → motor nucleus of N. V → jaw closing |
| Nerve VII | taste-salivary reflex | the presence of salivation following application of a taste stimulus on the tongue: afferent SVA fibers of N. VII → solitary nucleus → superior and inferior salivatory nuclei → parasympathetic fibers to salivary glands → salivation |

| Nerves IX & X | carotid sinus (baro)reflex | sudden increase in blood pressure is followed by slowing of heart rate: baroreceptors in carotid sinus (N. IX) → solitary nucleus → dorsal motor nucleus of N. X → vagus nerve to heart → slowing of heart rate |
|---|---|---|
| Nerve IX | carotid body (chemoreceptor) reflex | higher levels of $CO_2$ in blood leads to inspiratory movements which lower $CO_2$ levels and increase $O_2$ levels: chemoreceptors in carotid body sense increased levels of $CO_2$ → N. IX → reticular formation of medulla → reticulospinal fibers to thoracic cord → phrenic and intercostal nerves → muscles of diaphragm → inspiration. (This response is terminated when inflated lung stimulates afferent fibers in vagus nerve → solitary nucleus and related neurons in reticular formation → inhibition of descending reticulospinal neurons that caused inspiratory responses to take place.) |
| Nerves IX & X | gag reflex | stimulation of the region of the pharynx results in elevation and contraction of pharynx: afferent fibers in N. IX → (possibly to solitary nucleus) or directly to → nucleus ambiguus of N. IX and N. X → muscles of the pharynx and palate |
| Nerve X | cough reflex | irritation of the larynx (or possibly other parts of the respiratory system such as trachea and bronchi) results in coughing: irritation → afferent impulses in N. X → solitary nucleus and reticular formation. The solitary nucleus → n. ambiguus → pharynx and larynx muscles to produce coughing movements. The reticular formation → to regions of the medulla that regulate expiratory responses (that comprise part of the coughing reflex) |

## SENSORY SYSTEMS

19. Loss of partial or total aspects of the visual field can be understood in terms of damage to the retinal pathways, including their targets in the lateral geniculate nucleus and visual cortex. The schematic diagram shown below depicts the kinds of field deficits that occur following lesions of different aspects of the visual pathway. Key: (A) optic nerve lesion producing total blindness in left eye; (B) lesion that disrupts right retinal nasal fibers that project from base of left optic nerve producing right upper quadrantanopia and left scotoma; (C) lesion of optic chiasm producing bitemporal hemianopia; (D) unilateral (left) optic tract lesion producing a right homonymous hemianopia; (E) interruption of left visual radiations that pass ventrally through temporal lobe to lower bank of visual cortex (i.e., loop of Meyer) producing an upper right quadrantanopia; (F) interruption of left visual radiations that pass more dorsally through the occipital lobe to the upper bank of visual cortex, producing a lower right quadrantanopia; and (G) lesion of left visual cortex that produces a

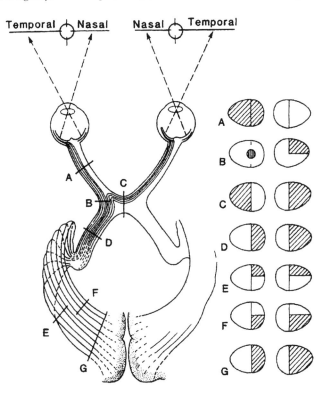

right homonymous hemianopsia. (Adams et al., Principles of Neurology, 1997, McGraw-Hill, with permission of the McGraw-Hill Companies).

20. Key principles underlying sensory functions: (1) excitatory focus and surround inhibition; and (2) somatotopic organization. These are present within a given receptor system and form the functional basis for discriminative functions in a number of the sensory systems, including the auditory circuit.

    Auditory pathways—complex and involve the following synaptic connections: first-order root fibers of the spiral ganglion (originate in organ of Corti of cochlea) → cochlear nuclei of upper medulla → via lateral lemniscus → inferior colliculus → medial geniculate nucleus → superior temporal gyrus (primary auditory cortex).

21. Vestibular pathway: first-order neurons originate from vestibular ganglion and have peripheral processes located in specialized receptors in utricle, saccule and semicircular canals. The central branches of this neuron → vestibular nuclei → cerebellar cortex (Flocculonodular lobe) or via medial longitudinal fasciculus rostrally or caudally →NIII, IV, or VI of the midbrain and pons or spinal cord, respectively. Damage to these fibers, especially within the medial longitudinal fasciculus or cerebellum, produces nystagmus (i.e., involuntary movement of the eyes, in the horizontal or vertical plane, first slowly and then followed by a rapid jerking return).

## MOTOR SYSTEMS

22. (A) Voluntary motor control affecting mainly the flexor system: expressed through the descending pyramidal tracts plus the rubrospinal tract, while control of functions associated with posture is mediated through such descending pathways as the vestibulo- and reticulo-spinal tracts.

23. Modulation of motor functions is mediated by the basal ganglia and cerebellum. Involuntary motor disturbances at rest (called dyskinesias) are associated with the disruption of functions of the basal ganglia, while motor disturbances occurring during attempts at movement are frequently associated with damage to the cerebellum or its afferent or efferent pathways.

    A. The basal ganglia: consists of the neostriatum (caudate nucleus and putamen), paleostriatum (globus pallidus), and two additional structures that are anatomically and functionally related to the basal ganglia: the substantia nigra and subthalamic nucleus.

       (1) The following disorders are associated with damage to different parts of the basal ganglia: Parkinson's disease, chorea, athetosis, hemiballism, and tardive dyskinesia.

    B. The cerebellum consists of three lobes: anterior, posterior and flocculonodular lobes. The hemispheres of each lobe are by a medial vermal region.

**Table VII**
**Upper Motor Neurons**

| Pathway | Origin | Afferent Sources | Distribution | Function | Lesion Effects |
|---|---|---|---|---|---|
| Lateral Cortico-spinal tract | precentral, postcentral, supplementary and premotor cortices | basal ganglia, cerebellum to areas 4 and 6; somatosensory to areas 3,1,2 and precentral gyrus; posterior parietal cortex to area 6 | to all levels of contralateral spinal cord; areas 4 and 6 to ventral horn cells; areas 3,1,2 to dorsal horn | voluntary control of movements and sequencing of responses | upper motoneuron paralysis of contralateral limb; spasticity; hypertonia; positive Babinski sign; lesion of areas 5, 7, and 6 produce apraxia |
| Cortico-bulbar tract | precentral (lateral aspect), postcentral (lateral aspect) | somatosensory from trigeminal afferents | to cranial nerve motor nuclei; bilateral except for nerves VII (neurons that innervate lower jaw muscles) and XII; corti-co-reticular; and corti-corubral fibers | voluntary control of motor functions of the face; inputs to reticular formation provide another mechanism by which cortex regulates spinal motor functions | some weakness of the affected muscles except for lower jaw muscles and tongue which are deviated to the opposite side; loss of cortical inputs to reticular formation may account for spasticity in upper motoneuron disorder |

| Tract | Source | Inputs | Projection | Function | Lesion effects |
|---|---|---|---|---|---|
| Rubrospinal tract | Red nucleus | motor and premotor cortices project somatotopically to the red nucleus; inputs from cerebellum | cells in dorsal region project to contralateral cervical levels; cells in ventral region project to contralateral lumbar cord | facilitates flexor motor neuron; functions as a parallel pathway to the corticospinal tract | difficult to assess because pure lesions of the red nucleus are rarely if ever found; ataxia and oculomotor palsy (Benedikt's syndrome) may be attributed to other pathways such as cerebellar efferents and N. III |
| Lateral Reticulospinal tract | medial two thirds of medulla (n. reticularis gigantocellularis) | motor and premotor cortices | project to spinal cord in ventral funiculus; innervates ventral horn cells; acts mainly on extensors | inhibits spinal motor neuron activity; particular emphasis on gamma efferents and muscle tone | specific effects are unclear; but loss of input from cortex or damage to pathway will likely produce spasticity and hypertonicity |
| Medial Reticulospinal tract | medial two thirds of pons (n. reticularis pontis oralis and caudalis) | motor and premotor cortices; sensory inputs from ascending pathways | project to spinal cord in ventral funiculus; innervates ventral horn cells; acts mainly on extensors | facilitates spinal reflexes, especially those of extensors; particular emphasis upon gamma motor neuron, increase muscle tone | unclear; specific lesion data is unavailable; it may be suggested that lesions would increase likelihood of hypotonicity and hyperreflexia |

**Table VII (Cont.)**

| Pathway | Origin | Afferent Sources | Distribution | Function | Lesion Effects |
|---|---|---|---|---|---|
| Lateral Vestibulo-spinal tract | lateral vestibular nucleus | vestibular apparatus and cerebellum | projects to all levels of spinal cord in ventral funiculus | powerfully facilitates spinal motor neurons that innervate extensors | data unavailable, but likely would produce diminution of effectiveness of antigravity muscles and muscle tone in those muscles |
| Medial Vestibulo-spinal tract | medial vestibular nucleus | vestibular apparatus | projects mainly to cervical cord, in particular to spinal accessory nucleus | modulates actions of motor neurons of the accessory nerve; head turning and lifting of head, in particular in response to stimulation of the labyrinth | data unavailable; but a lesion would probably disrupt reflex actions between changes in posture and appropriate adjustment of head in response to stimulation of the labyrinth |
| Tectospinal tract | superior colliculus | retinal fibers | projection to contralateral cervical cord; fibers contained in anterior funiculus | provides postural reflex adjustments in response to visual stimuli | unknown |

**Table VIII**

Inputs, Internal and Output Circuitry of the Basal Ganglia

| Structure | afferent | Transmitter | Function | Efferent | Transmitter | Function |
|---|---|---|---|---|---|---|
| *Neostriatum* | cerebral cortex, centromedian n. | glutamate | excites neostriatal neurons | 1) globus pallidus (med.) 2) globus pallidus (lat.) 3) substantia nigra (pars reticulata) | GABA to globus pallidus (med.) GABA and enkephalin to globus pallidus (lat.) GABA to substantia nigra (pars reticulata) | inhibition of neurons in both medial and lateral segments of the globus pallidus; inhibition of neurons in substantia nigra (pars reticulata) |
| | | acetylcholine | excitatory neurotransmitter for interneurons within the neostriatum | | | |
| *Globus pallidus (lateral)* | neostriatum | GABA, enkephalin | inhibition of pallidal neurons | subthalamic nucleus | GABA | inhibition of subthalamic neurons |

**Table VIII (Cont.)**

| Structure | afferent | Transmitter | Function | Efferent | Transmitter | Function |
|---|---|---|---|---|---|---|
| *Globus pallidus (medial)* | neostriatum, subthalamic nucleus | GABA (from neostriatum) glutamate (from subthalamic nucleus) | inhibition of pallidal neurons by the neostriatum; excitation of pallidal neurons by the subthalamic nucleus | ventrolateral, ventral anterior and centro-median nuclei of thalamus | GABA | inhibition of thalamic neurons that project to motor regions of cortex |
| *Subthalamic nucleus* | globus pallidus (lateral) | GABA | inhibition of subthalamic neurons | globus pallidus (medial) | glutamate | excitation of neurons of medial pallidal segment |
| *Substantia nigra (pars compacta)* | substantia nigra (pars reticulata) | GABA? | inhibition of neurons in pars compacta | neostriatum | dopamine | excitation of neostriatal neurons that project to the globus pallidus (medial); inhibition of neurons that project to the globus pallidus (lateral) |

| Substantia nigra (pars reticulata) | neostriatum | GABA and substance P | GABA-inhibition of reticulata neurons; substance P - excitation of reticulata neurons | ventrolateral and ventral anterior nuclei of thalamus; superior colliculus | GABA<br><br>Substance P | inhibition of thalamic neurons that project to motor regions of cortex; reflex control of eye movements |

## Table IX
## Diseases of the Basal Ganglia

| Disease | Lesion | Changes in in Transmitter | Symptom | Comment |
|---|---|---|---|---|
| *Parkinson's disease* | Destruction of cells in pars compacta of substantia nigra and of nigral striatal pathway | Reduction in striatal dopamine; also loss of norepinephrine and serotonin elsewhere in the brain | tremor at rest, rigidity, bradykinesia, akinesia | Some success with L-dopa and anticholinergic drug therapy; lesions of the ventrolateral nucleus have also shown some success; transplantation of dopaminergic cells into neostriatum is in experimental stages; some success with surgical lesions of the medial pallidal segment and with electrical stimulation of subthalamic nucleus |
| *Chorea (Huntington's Disease)* | damage to neurons in the neostriatum (includes GABA and cholinergic cells) | reduction of striatal GABA and acetylcholine | Wild, uncontrolled, abrupt and jerky movements of the distal musculature; Huntington's disease—genetic effect located on short arm of chromosome 4; autosomal dominant | Loss of inhibition onto subthalamic nucleus because of damage to inhibitory (GABAergic) projections from neostriatum to the lateral pallidal segment; net result is loss of inhibitory ... from pallidum |

| | | | |
|---|---|---|---|
| **Hemiballism** | discrete damage to neurons in the subthalamic nucleus | possible loss of glutamate in subthalamic nucleus | involuntary ballistic movement of limb contralateral to the lesion | onto thalamus, thus causing excess movement from cortex; administration of dopamine antagonists and phenothiazines are sometimes helpful  The only disorder of the basal ganglia for which a specific locus has been identified |
| **Athetosis** and **dystonia** | neostriatum (and possibly cerebral cortex as well) | probable loss of GABA and acetylcholine | slow, writhing involuntary movements of the extremities | Dystonia: when athetoid movements involve the axial musculature of the neck and shoulder girdle, and are sustained, they frequently cause twisting and repetitive movements or abnormal postures |
| **Tardive dyskinesia** | dopamine receptor blockade in neostriatum | dopamine receptor blockade in neostriatum causes hypersensitivity to dopamine and agonists of dopamine | involuntary movements of the tongue and face | Disorder is induced, not by lesions, but by antipsychotic drugs that block dopaminergic transmission; disorder can be stopped by eliminating drugs that induced this response pattern |

## Table X
## Afferent Connections of the Cerebellum

| Pathway | Origin | Peduncle | Region of termination | Function |
|---|---|---|---|---|
| **Spinal Cord:** | | | | |
| (1) dorsal spinocerebellar tract | n. dorsalis of Clarke (C8-L3) | ICP | anterior lobe | conveys muscle spindle and Golgi tendon organ inputs from lower limb |
| (2) ventral spinocerebellar tract | scattered cells near ventral horn of lumbar/thoracic cord | SCP | anterior lobe (vermal region) | conveys Golgi tendon organ inputs from lower limb |
| (3) cuneocerebellar tract | accessory cuneate nucleus | ICP | anterior lobe | conveys muscle spindle and Golgi tendon organ inputs from upper limb |
| (4) rostral spinocerebellar tract | cervical cord | ICP and SCP | anterior lobe | conveys Golgi tendon organ inputs from upper limb (found in cat only) |
| **Brainstem:** | | | | |
| (1) olivo-cerebellar fibers | inferior olivary nucleus: afferents to inferior olivary n. from spinal cord, red n. and cerebral cortex | ICP | anterior and posterior lobes | conveys flexor reflex and cutaneous afferents from spinal cord and inputs from red nucleus to cerebellar cortex |
| (2) vestibulo-cerebellar fibers | primary vestibular neurons and vestibular nuclei | ICP | flocculonodular lobe | conveys vestibular inputs to cerebellum |

| | | | | |
|---|---|---|---|---|
| (3) reticulo-cerebellar fibers | reticular nuclei of medulla and pons and afferents from cerebral cortex | ICP and MCP | anterior and posterior lobes | provides cerebellar cortex with information concerning the status of reticular neurons that modulate the gamma motor system |
| (4) trigemino-cerebellar fibers | mesencephalic n. of N. V (spinal n.) | MCP and ICP | vermal and paravermal regions of anterior and posterior lobes | mediates muscle spindle and some tactile inputs to cerebellar cortex |
| (5) aminergic fibers | raphe nucleus and locus ceruleus | MCP | wide areas of cerebellar cortex | modulates activity of cerebellar cortical neurons, and in particular, those of Purkinje cells |
| (6) tecto-cerebellar fibers | superior and inferior colliculi | MCP | vermal and paravermal region of anterior and posterior lobes | mediates auditory and visual signals to cerebellar cortex; possibly contributes to the process of learning within cerebellum |
| (7) ponto-cerebellar fibers | deep pontine nuclei—receives major inputs from cerebral cortex | MCP | topographic distribution to hemispheres of anterior and posterior lobes | provides inputs to cerebellar cortex from all parts of the cerebral cortex—important for the initiation and planning of movement |

ICP, inferior cerebellar peduncle; MCP, middle cerebellar peduncle; SCP, superior cerebellar peduncle

## Table XI
### Efferent Connections of the Cerebellum

| Deep Cerebellar Nucleus | Afferent Connection | Efferent Connection | Function |
|---|---|---|---|
| fastigial nucleus | vermal region of cerebellar cortex | vestibular nuclei and reticular formation of medulla and pons | part of feedback circuit mediating control of postural mechanisms and muscle tone |
| interposed nuclei | paravermal and intermediate region of cerebellar cortex | red nucleus via superior cerebellar peduncle | part of feedback circuit mediating control of flexor motor system and overall regulation of the distal musculature |
| dentate nucleus | lateral regions of cerebellar hemisphere | ventrolateral nucleus of thalamus via superior cerebellar peduncle | mediates signals to cerebral cortex for initiation and programming of motor sequences |

(2) Disorders of the cerebellum typically occur when movement is attempted.

## Table XII
### Regional Localization of Cerebellar Disorders

| Lobe of Cerebellum | Disorder Resulting from Lesion |
|---|---|
| Anterior lobe (paleocerebellum) | characterized by a wide, staggering gait ataxia resulting primarily from damage affecting the vermal and paravermal regions |
| Posterior lobe (neocerebellum) | characterized by loss of coordination while executing voluntary movements |
| Flocculonodular lobe (archicerebellum) | characterized by a loss of equilibrium with the patient displaying a wide, staggering ataxic gait. Lesions of this region also produce eye movement disorders, including nystagmus |

# HIGHER AUTONOMIC AND BEHAVIORAL FUNCTIONS

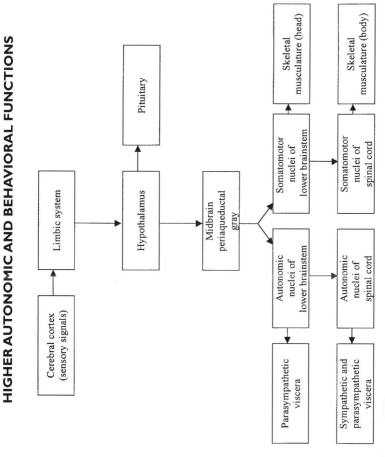

24. As shown on p. 259, autonomic, endocrine and emotional functions are mediated by the limbic system (when activated by sensory inputs from the cerebral cortex), hypothalamus, and midbrain periaqueductal gray matter: (a) emotional behavior and autonomic functions: limbic structures (hippocampal formation, septal area, amygdala, anterior cingulate gyrus, prefrontal cortex) → hypothalamus → midbrain periaqueductal gray → autonomic neurons in lower medulla and somatomotor neurons of brainstem (i.e., cranial nerve nuclei for expression of motor aspects of emotional behavior) → autonomic and somatomotor neurons of the spinal cord; and (b) regulation of endocrine functions: limbic structures to: → (1) supraoptic and paraventricular nuclei of hypothalamus → posterior lobe of pituitary; and (2) medial hypothalamus → anterior lobe of pituitary (via vascular system).

**Properties of these neurons:** (I) Limbic projections to hypothalamus modulate endocrine functions of the hypothalamus; (II) disruption of hypothalamic neurons alters rage behavior, temperature regulation, sexual behavior, feeding, drinking, and endocrine functions; damage to limbic neurons frequently lead to temporal lobe epilepsy, produce short-term memory deficits (especially with hippocampal damage); and alter threshold for the expression of rage behavior (e.g., Klüver-Bucy syndrome)

## Table XIII
### Hypothalamic Nuclei: Input-Output Relationships

| Structure | Afferent Source(s) | Efferent Projections | Functions |
|---|---|---|---|
| preoptic region | medial amygdala subfornical organ | median eminence; posterior pituitary | regulates heat loss; drinking; regulation of sleep |
| supraoptic nucleus | subfornical organ | posterior pituitary; median eminence | antidiuretic hormone (oxytocin) release |
| paraventricular nucleus | limbic structures subfornical organ | posterior pituitary; median eminence; autonomic nuclei of lower brainstem | oxytocin and antidiuretic hormone release; regulation of sympathetic activity |
| suprachiasmatic nucleus | retinal fibers; hippocampal formation (fornix) | paraventricular nucleus to autonomic nuclei of lower brainstem | control of circadian rhythms for sex hormones, corticosterone, melatonin, and sleep |

| lateral hypothalamus | limbic structures: (basal amygdala, hippocampal formation through septal nuclei, pre-frontal cortex through medial thalamus and midline nuclei); brainstem reticular formation and monoamine neurotransmitters | periaqueductal gray and other parts of midbrain tegmentum, locus ceruleus and motor nucleus of N. V; feedback projections to the septal area; lateral habenular nucleus through stria medullaris | feeding behavior; predatory attack behavior in the cat |
|---|---|---|---|
| medial hypothalamus | medial amygdala; bed nucleus of stria terminalis; septal area | dorsal half of midbrain periaqueductal gray | defensive rage behavior in the cat; sexual behavior (lordosis); inhibition of feeding ; sympathetic activation |
| posterior hypothalamus | anterior hypothalamus; brainstem reticular formation and monoamine fibers | autonomic nuclei of the lower brainstem | heat conservation; sympathetic activation |
| mammillary bodies | hippocampal formation (fornix) | anterior thalamic nucleus (mammillo-thalamic tract); midbrain tegmentum (mammillotegmental tract) | generally unknown but may participate in memory functions with other parts of Papez circuit |

## Table XIV
## Hypothalamic Relationships with the Pituitary Gland

| Hormone | Location (cell body) | Terminal Region | Function |
|---|---|---|---|
| *Posterior pituitary:* | | | |
| antidiuretic hormone | supraoptic, paraventricular nuclei | posterior pituitary | promotes water reabsorption from distal convoluted tubules |
| oxytocin | paraventricular and supraoptic nuclei | posterior pituitary | aids in milk ejection reflex and causes uterine contractions at birth |
| *Anterior pituitary:* | | | |
| growth hormone releasing hormone (GHrH) | arcuate nucleus | median eminence | stimulates release of growth hormone |
| somatostatin | preoptic region and anterior hypothalamus | median eminence | inhibits growth hormone (also thyrotropin and prolactin) |
| thyrotropin releasing hormone | periventricular region | median eminence | stimulates release of thyroid stimulating hormone |
| corticotropin releasing hormone | paraventricular, supraoptic and arcuate nuclei | median eminence | stimulates release of adrenocorticotrophic hormone (ACTH) |
| gonadotropin releasing hormone | most dense in arcuate region but found elsewhere in hypothalamus | median eminence | stimulates release of follicle stimulating hormone and luteinizing hormone |
| prolactin releasing factor | periventricular region? | median eminence | stimulates release of prolactin |
| dopamine | arcuate region | median eminence | inhibits prolactin release |

**Table XV**
**Other Hypothalamic Peptides and Their Functions**

| Peptide | Location (cell body) | Function |
|---|---|---|
| vasoactive intestinal peptide (VIP) | suprachiasmatic nucleus, anterior pituitary (and cerebral cortex) | modulates activity of suprachiasmatic nucleus and release of anterior pituitary hormones |
| cholecystokinin (CCK-8) | posterior pituitary, supraoptic, and paraventricular nuclei | modulates release of oxytocin and vasopressin from hypothalamic nuclei; also inhibits feeding behavior |
| neurotensin | preoptic area, anterior and dorsomedial hypothalamus | modulates release of pituitary hormones and possibly release of dopamine into portal system |
| enkephalins | found widely in CNS | inhibits endocrine and non-endocrine functions of hypothalamus |
| angiotensin II | supraoptic and paraventricular region | regulates blood pressure; induces drinking behavior |
| substance P | medial amygdala, anterior hypothalamus with terminals and receptors in medial hypothalamus | facilitates functions of the medial hypothalamus such as defensive rage and possibly sexual behavior |
| galanin | paraventricular region | induces feeding |
| neuropeptide Y | widely distributed in CNS and hypothalamus | modulates GnRH containing neurons (i.e., gonadotropin secretion) |
| endothelin | supraoptic and paraventricular regions | increases LH secretion by stimulating GnRH containing neurons |

**Table XVI**
**Structures of the Limbic System and Their Functions**

| Structure | Afferent Fibers | Efferent Fibers | Functions | Effects of Lesions |
|---|---|---|---|---|
| *Hippocampal formation* | (1) septal fibers contained in fornix; (2) tertiary sensory [olfactory, visual, auditory] afferents from entorhinal cortex; (3) cingulate cortex afferent fibers; (4) monoaminergic fibers; (5) some posterior hypothalamic afferent fibers | (1) postcommissural fornix (from subicular cortex) to mammillary bodies, anterior thalamic nucleus and ventromedial hypothalamus; (2) precommissural fornix (from CA fields and subiculum) to septal area; (3) to entorhinal cortex and amygdala | modulation of hypothalamic functions (aggression and rage, endocrine functions); short-term memory functions; role in the genesis of epilepsy | temporal lobe epilepsy; rage and aggressive behavior; short-term memory disorders |
| *Septal area* | (1) fornix fibers from hippocampal formation; (2) monoaminergic fibers from brainstem; (3) lateral hypothalamic afferents in medial forebrain bundle; (4) medial olfactory stria (secondary olfactory signals) | (1) lateral septal efferents through medial forebrain bundle to hypothalamus; (2) medial septal-diagonal band efferents to hippocampal formation; (3) diagonal band efferents to cortex, medial thalamus, mammillary bodies | similar to hippocampal formation (modulation of hypothalamic functions); serves as a relay for hippocampal inputs to hypothalamus | septal rage in rats; alterations in visceral functions normally associated with hypothalamus |
| *Amygdala* | (1) olfactory, taste, and auditory inputs from | (1) corticomedial amygdala via stria | powerful modulation of rage and aggression; | temporal lobe epilepsy; fits of rage and aggres- |

| | | | | |
|---|---|---|---|---|
| | lateral olfactory stria, solitary nucleus, and temporal neocortex, respectively; (2) monoaminergic inputs from brainstem; (3) from subicular cortex; (4) from prefrontal cortex | terminalis to medial hypothalamus; (2) basolateral amygdala via ventral amygdalofugal pathway to lateral hypothalamus and midbrain periaqueductal gray; (3) projections from wide regions of amygdala to the bed nucleus of stria terminalis | regulation of feeding, drinking, endocrine and cardiovascular functions associated with the hypothalamus and midbrain periaqueductal gray | sion; alterations in feeding, drinking, autonomic and endocrine functions |
| *Prefrontal cortex* | (1) all regions of neocortex; (2) mediodorsal thalamic nucleus; (3) monoaminergic brainstem fibers; (4) limbic nuclei—subicular cortex, diagonal band nuclei, and lateral hypothalamus [including substantia innominata] | (1) mediodorsal thalamic nucleus [and through additional interneurons in midline thalamus to anterior lateral hypothalamus]; (2) to limbic structures—subicular cortex and amygdala | powerful regulation of aggression, rage and autonomic functions of the hypothalamus; intellectual functions; mood states | intellectual and perceptual deficits; marked personality and mood changes as well as alterations in ability to regulate autonomic functions |
| *Anterior cingulate cortex* | (1) anterior nucleus of thalamus; (2) nuclei of diagonal band of Broca; (3) dopaminergic fibers from ventral tegmental area | (1) mediodorsal thalamic nucleus; (2) presubiculum | (1) regulation of rage and aggression and other autonomic functions associated with the hypothalamus | changes in emotional behavior, personality and mood states |

## Table XVI (Cont.)

| Structure | Afferent Fibers | Efferent Fibers | Functions | Effects of Lesions |
|---|---|---|---|---|
| *Limbic forebrain nuclei:* | | | | |
| *(1) bed nucleus of stria terminalis* | amygdaloid nuclei; brainstem monoaminergic nuclei; hypothalamus | hypothalamus and midbrain periaqueductal gray | regulation of aggression and rage and autonomic functions | unknown |
| *(2) nucleus accumbens* | subicular cortex; brainstem monoaminergic nuclei | ventral tegmental area; substantia innominata | integration of motor and limbic processes | unknown |
| *(3) substantia innominata (basal nucleus of Meynert)* | amygdala; brainstem monoaminergic nuclei | lateral hypothalamus; limbic structures; wide regions of cortex | related to sleep-wakefulness cycle; learning and memory functions of the cortex; regulation of rage, aggression and autonomic functions of the hypothalamus | damage to the basal nucleus of Meynert has been associated with cholinergic reductions in neocortex and Alzheimer's disease |

# CEREBRAL CORTEX

25. Dysfunctions associated with cerebrovascular accidents and tumors can be understood in terms of the principles of cortical localization and cerebral dominance. The table below lists common disorders, their descriptions, and the cortical regions most closely associated with each disorder.

## Table XVII
### Upper Motor Neurons

| Disease | Affected Structure(s) | Description of Loss |
|---|---|---|
| Upper motor neuron paralysis | Precentral, premotor and supplemental motor areas (as well as internal capsule, crus cerebri, or corticospinal tracts) | Loss of voluntary control of upper and lower limbs (depending upon extent of lesion); this disorder is also associated with hyperreflexia, hypertonicity and a positive Babinski sign |
| Broca's aphasia | Inferior frontal gyrus of dominant hemisphere | Patient cannot name simple objects but has no difficulty in comprehending spoken language |
| Wernicke's aphasia | Superior temporal gyrus and adjoining regions | Patient has difficulty in comprehending language but speech appears fluent |
| Astereognosia | Parietal cortex | Failure of tactile recognition of objects (e.g., blackboard eraser, pack of cigarettes) on side contralateral to lesion |
| Unilateral sensory neglect | Parietal cortex (usually of right hemisphere) | Patient ignores stimuli on opposite (i.e., left) side of body space, which includes visual, somatosensory and auditory stimuli. Examples: patient neglects to shave side of face contralateral to lesion and will deny that there is anything wrong with that side of body even if there is a motor paralysis. Patient may further draw a picture of flowers or of a clock in which petals on flowers or numbers on clock are limited to right side of each of the figures |

## Table XVII (Cont.)

| Disease | Affected Structure(s) | Description of Loss |
|---------|----------------------|---------------------|
| Apraxia | Posterior parietal cortex | Patient is unable to conceptualize sequence of events necessary to carry out a task even though basic sensory and motor pathways necessary to produce required movements are intact. |

# BIBLIOGRAPHY

Adams RD, Victor M, Ropper, AH: *Principles of Neurology*, 6/e. New York, McGraw-Hill, 1997.

Carpenter MB, Sutin J: *Human Neuroanatomy*, 8/e. Baltimore, Williams & Wilkins, 1983.

Cooper JR, Bloom FE, Roth RH: *The Biochemical Basis of Neuropharmacology*, 7/e. New York, Oxford University Press, 1996.

DeArmond SJ, Fusco MM, Dewey MM: *Structure of the Human Brain: A Photographic Atlas*, 3/e. New York, Oxford University Press, 1989.

Guyton AC: *Basic Neuroscience: Anatomy and Physiology*, 2/e. Philadelphia, Saunders, 1991.

Haines DE (Ed.): *Fundamental Neuroscience*, New York, Churchill Livingstone, 1997.

Kandel ER, Schwartz JH, Jessel TM: *Principles of Neural Science*, 3/e. New York, Elsevier, 1991.

Rowland LP (Ed.): *Merritt's Textbook of Neurology*, 9/e. Baltimore, Williams & Wilkins, 1995.

Noback CR, Strominger NL, Demarest RJ: *The Human Nervous System*, 5/e. Baltimore, Williams & Wilkins, 1996.

Siegel GJ, Agranoff BW, Albers RW, Molinoff PB: *Basic Neurochemistry*, 5/e. New York, Raven, 1994.

Villiger E, Ludwig E, Rasmussen AT: *Atlas of Cross Section Anatomy of the Brain*. New York, McGraw-Hill, 1951.

Wilson-Pauwels L, Akesson EJ, Stewart PA: *Cranial Nerves: Gross Anatomy and Clinical Comments*. Toronto, Decker, 1988.

ISBN 0-07-052690-7

9 780070 526907

90000

SIEGEL: NEUROSCIENCE